ISBN: 1453731806
ISBN-13: 9781453731802
Library of Congress Control Number: 2010914467

Stem Cells 4 U?

What Stem Cells Can Really Do
—
Now and in the Future

Hans Klingemann, MD, PhD

To my wife Sandra for her insightful
support and encouragement

To our patients who are waiting for answers

CONTENTS

PREFACE

Why a book about stem cells? Because there is so much enthusiasm about their potential at all levels of our society, but there is also so much misinformation about stem cells in the news media, blogs, social sites, and in advertisements. These reports raise the hopes of patients who may be desperately looking for effective stem cell therapies. However, the true advances in stem cell medicine may go unnoticed because they are not deemed as newsworthy, are not as attractive to investors, or are not relevant to political advances.

Although the potential of stem cells for tissue engineering and regenerative medicine is very real and promising, it is often ignored that for decades, cancer specialists have been performing bone marrow stem cell transplants using adult stem cells, initially from siblings and later also from unrelated volunteer donors or umbilical cord blood. Among the many diseases that can now be treated with a bone marrow stem cell transplant, leukemia, lymphoma, myeloma, bone marrow failure, metabolic disorders, and immune deficiencies are the most common. This book tells the stories of patients whose lives have been transformed by this remarkable procedure.

This text is not meant to teach the reader about stem cells in a scholarly way. Rather, it will explain the relevance of the different stem cells in the context of potential clinical applications. The ultimate goal of this book is to provide unbiased and easy to follow information to you, the interested reader, the patient, the concerned parent, or even the curious investor to be better positioned to identify credible medical progress and what it holds for the future.

It is likely that stem cells particularly for regenerative medicine will become more widely available for patients in the near future. They are already used for bone and cartilage replacement, and to support the healing of wounds. They have also entered the field of veterinary medicine. At the end of the text active clinical trials are listed that are conducted with stem cells in North America, most of which have the approval of the Federal Drug Administration (FDA). There is a plethora of stem cell treatments offered at clinics and hospitals abroad. Anecdotal patient testimonies and the buildup of hope in desperate patients have resulted in the creation of a new medical industry with great potential but limited factual perspective.

The author's career as a stem cell transplant physician and scientist on the forefront of this medical revolution has afforded him the opportunity to talk to numerous patients and laymen about this topic and learn the importance of presenting this complex field balanced and easy to comprehend.

For more detailed information on stem cells, the Web sites of the National Institutes of Health (www.stemcells.nih.gov/info/basics) or the National Academy of Sciences (www.nationalacademies.org/stemcells) are recommended.

I.

DIAGNOSIS LEUKEMIA: KATE NEEDS A BONE MARROW STEM CELL TRANSPLANT

Kate, her husband, Mark, and their two children, Anna-Maria and Christopher, were driving home to Boston on a Sunday night after a long weekend on Cape Cod. Kate had been feeling tired for a couple of weeks and had noticed some blood stains on her tooth brush, which she assumed were from some mild gum bleeds. She was too busy with her job and her family to pay much attention to her symptoms. When she continued to feel easily exhausted, and friends continued to mention to her that she looked a bit pale lately, she finally called Dr. Phillips, her primary care physician. He thought that she might have had a bout with the flu but suggested running some blood tests, including a complete blood count or CBC. A CBC measures the number of red blood cells (which carry oxygen), the number of platelets (which are important for proper blood clotting), and the number of white blood cells (which fight infection). Kate had blood drawn in the physician's office, and Christine, one of her physician's nurses telephoned her with the results.

Christine told her that her CBC was abnormal; she had a low number of red cells and platelets, and her white cell count was quite high—five times higher than what is considered normal. She told Kate to come back to the office because Dr. Phillips wanted to talk to her. Dr. Phillips saw Kate right away when she arrived at his office. He looked concerned and explained that she needed to see a hematologist, a specialist who handles blood and bone marrow disorders. Dr. Phillips exclaimed, "This is urgent, and you need to be seen right away!" He also told her that a bone marrow biopsy would likely be needed to find out what kind of bone marrow disease was causing her abnormal blood results. When Kate asked him what this could mean, his reply was a bit vague, but he hinted that it could be a form of leukemia that would need to be treated urgently.

Kate scheduled an appointment with the hematologist Dr. Sullivan for that afternoon. As Dr. Phillips had warned, Dr. Sullivan told her that a bone marrow biopsy was needed, and the procedure was done right in his office. The biopsy is a relatively minor procedure that is performed whenever there is suspicion of a bone marrow or blood disorder. The patient lies on her stomach or on the side, and the physician uses a needle to go into the hipbone. Kate was given some intravenous medication to make her more relaxed and provide some pain relief. Dr. Sullivan also took some time to numb the puncture site with a local anesthetic to minimize any pain. While the procedure took only a few minutes and even with the numbing, it was a bit painful, especially when Dr. Sullivan applied a sucking pressure with the syringe to extract the bone marrow.

The nurse put some of the sample on a glass slide to confirm that it contained actual marrow and not just blood. This sample can be evaluated by the hematologist right away under a regular microscope and can often provide an early diagnosis. The remainder of the bone marrow sample was sent for special studies: one to evaluate the chromosomes or genetic makeup of the cells and the other to evaluate the surface of the cells. It can take up to two weeks to receive results from these tests, but they can help the physician understand exactly what type of leukemia, if any, is present and how likely it is to respond to treatment. After this was done, Dr. Sullivan performed the second part of the procedure. He carved out a small cone from the bone, maybe half an inch in length that was also sent to the pathologist. The review of the biopsy material usually takes a few days because the bone structures need to be dissolved in a special chemical to expose the cells. The pathologist can tell whether there are leukemia cells (known as *blasts*) and if so, how much of the bone marrow space is taken up by these cells.

Kate did not have to wait long. Dr. Sullivan phoned her the next day and asked her to come back to the office to talk about the result of the bone marrow biopsy. The marrow samples he examined under the microscope were sufficient to make the diagnosis. Kate wanted to know if they could talk over the phone about it, but he insisted that she see him in his office. Although Kate had planned a busy morning, she went in to talk to him.

"This is not good news" he began. "Your bone marrow biopsy has confirmed my most serious concern - you have leukemia, and you need treatment immediately." Hearing those words, Kate felt like she would faint. She knew what the diagnosis meant. One of her friends had died from complications of leukemia just last year after prolonged treatment. "What do you mean by immediate treatment?" she asked.

Dr. Sullivan explained, "Your white cell count is quite high, over fifty thousand. Normal is between four thousand and eight thousand. Such a high white cell count can cause problems, including difficulty breathing and in some cases even a stroke if the blood gets too "thick" from the high white cell count. Also, your platelet count is only fourteen thousand, and you are at risk for spontaneous hemorrhage. You need to be started on treatment today."

Kate was in shock, and her mind was racing. What would happen to her job? Who would take care of her children while she was getting the treatment? And most importantly, what were her prospects for the future?

Kate went directly to the hospital and was admitted to a special hematology unit. A needle was placed into her arm for intravenous fluid administration and more blood was drawn to run additional tests. She was given medication to combat nausea, a common side effect of chemotherapy, and then the chemotherapy was administered. Every day for the next seven days she received the *induction* phase of chemotherapy, which is intended to *induce* the disease into remission by killing the vast majority of the leukemic cells. Fortunately, she did not feel too nauseated, and although her appetite was not robust, she continued to eat. Her white cell count came down as expected. But along with the decline in bad leukemia cells, the few remaining normal white cells, which had protected her from getting an infection, were also dropping.

Three days after the chemotherapy infusions were finished, she developed a fever. An infection during this stage of chemotherapy is very serious since her immune system is unable to fight; antibiotics were started right away. Her appetite now was poor, and she needed intravenous nutrition that contained nutrients, vitamins, and minerals. The attending hematologist on the ward told her it would take about four weeks before her bone marrow would recover and start producing new blood cells again. She also needed another bone marrow biopsy two weeks into the therapy to make sure the treatment had killed all the leukemic cells.

Two weeks after learning that she had leukemia, Kate had a second bone marrow biopsy to determine if the chemotherapy was working. That biopsy showed that Kate's disease was in remission—finally some good news for her. Kate would be able to go home after her white cell count had recovered, which would probably be in another couple of weeks.

Although Kate had help from her mom, her lengthy hospitalization had been difficult for her husband and children. Unfortunately, she wasn't home for good—she would have to return to the hospital in three weeks for the *consolidation* phase of her chemotherapy. This is a second course of chemotherapy given over several days with the intent to eradicate or "mop up" any leukemic cells that may have survived the first induction phase of chemotherapy.

However, on the day of her expected admission, blood tests showed that Kate had some leukemia blasts circulating in her blood. Her leukemia had already come back—not a good sign. When leukemia returns so quickly, it is a sign of aggressive disease. Kate was devastated. The race against time had begun.

The treatment plans were changing. Instead of consolidation chemotherapy, Kate needed to repeat the induction phase of chemotherapy. That would again keep her in the hospital for at least another month.

But there was more. Kate was told she needed a bone marrow transplant—quickly. Her disease would not be controlled over the long-term period with just more chemotherapy. Even if her disease went back into remission, it was unlikely that it would stay in remission. Over time, her leukemia would actually learn how to survive the chemotherapy, rendering it ineffective (a process referred to as *resistance*). Kate needed healthy stem cells from another person to replace her diseased stem cells. The bone marrow transplant team at our hospital was called in.

Bone marrow stem cell transplants have been used for over fifty years to treat acute or chronic forms of leukemia, myelodysplastic syndrome (a precursor of acute leukemia), lymphoma (a cancerous growth of lymph nodes), and myeloma (a cancerous expansion of bone marrow plasma cells that can cause fractures and an elevation of a harmful protein in the blood). They are also used to treat non cancerous diseases like aplastic anemia, in which the bone marrow stops producing blood cells altogether. Although this disease is rarely seen in the United States today, it is still quite prevalent in certain parts of Asia and South America. Finally, there are several congenital metabolic disorders errors that can be cured by a bone marrow stem cell transplant. These disorders affect young children and result in the deposition of abnormal proteins in organs where they can impair their function.

Bone marrow contains a special type of adult stem cells that are responsible for producing different types of blood cells that carry oxygen (red cells or erythrocytes), fight infection (white cells or leukocytes), or can stop bleeding (platelets or thrombocytes). These bone marrow stem cells can give rise to different cell types that make up our blood and hence have been named *multipotent*. In contrast, *pluripotent* stem cells such as embryonic stem cells, can give rise to any type of cell found in the body. Both types of stem cells share the ability to self-renew and turn into different tissues.

Unfortunately it is impossible to pinpoint and localize stem cells in the bone marrow. They are inconspicuous in shape, size, and function, and they are present in very low numbers. Although physicians use a particular marker called CD34 that sticks out on the surface like a flag to identify them, CD34 captures only a small fraction of the adult stem cell population in the bone marrow.

II.
THE SEARCH FOR A STEM CELL DONOR

Because Kate's leukemia relapsed shortly after she had finished induction chemotherapy, a bone marrow or peripheral stem cell transplant was the only hope for her. Hematologists use these terms interchangeably, although the name *hematopoietic stem cell transplant* is more common and favored by many. Judy, our transplant coordinator, took a tube of blood from Kate the day tests revealed the relapse. The first step was to have her blood cells typed for her specific tissue markers and find out if she had a sibling who would match her tissue type.

The markers for tissue matching that transplant physicians are looking for are the *human leukocyte antigens* or HLA for short. These act like flags attached to body cells that signal the individuality of a person. They are the permanent makeup that all body cells carry. They help the cells of our immune system distinguish what is part of the body and protect from intruders such as bacteria, viruses, or cancer cells.

A complete tissue match between the bone marrow stem cells of the patient and the donor makes it less likely that the recipient will reject the transplanted bone marrow cells. A complete HLA match will also make it less likely that the transplanted donor cells will identify the patient's body cells as foreign and attack them. This latter reaction is essentially a reverse rejection and is called *graft versus host disease* (GvHD).

At birth, each of us receives two different sets of gene clusters from our parents, so there are four different combinations possible between siblings (figure 1). There is a twenty-five percent chance of finding a complete match among siblings. However, there can be families with seven or eight children in which there is no match, and families with only two children who happen to be HLA matched. Judy took the names and addresses of Kate's siblings. She would send them a kit in the mail that contained a plastic tube and a return envelope. They would take this to their primary care physician who would fill the tube with blood and send it back to Judy for HLA typing in the laboratory.

The HLA test tubes from Kate's siblings arrived a few weeks later, and we eagerly awaited the result. Unfortunately, none of Kate's siblings was a match. Kate's parents and children were also tested, but the chances of a patient having a tissue-matched parent or child, are extremely remote (< 1 percent), and some transplant centers don't even test parents or children. A match between parents and children can only occur when both parents, by a fluke, happen to share one set of chromosomes (a haplotype). Since none of Kate's siblings was matched, Kate's only chance now was to find an unrelated volunteer donor.

Since family size in our country is shrinking, chances of identifying a fully matched sibling are also declining. For that reason some transplant centers may accept siblings or relatives as donors who are not completely matched. However, this usually makes a transplant more risky, and complications after the transplant can be quite severe and longer lasting.

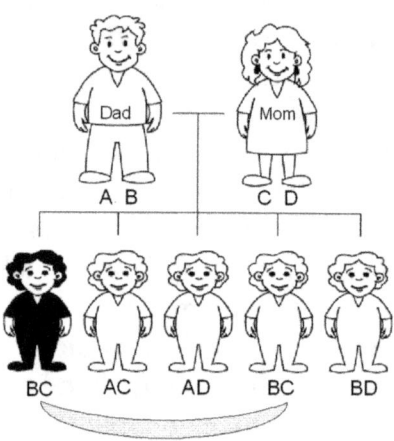

Figure 1

How the genes (chromosomes) and with them the individual tissue type is distributed and inherited within a family. Humans have forty-six chromosomes that carry our genes and are bundled in two sets of twenty-three each. One set is called a haplotype. Mom and Dad each have two different haplotypes (A and B, C and D) that are inherited separately. Hence four different haplotype combinations are possible among the children, and in this example, there is only one matched sibling pair, making the chances of finding a matched sibling in a family 25%.

THE NATIONAL MARROW DONOR PROGRAM (NMDP)

Since Kate did not have a perfect match in the family, the registry of the National Marrow Donor Program (NMDP) would have to be searched in the hope of finding a suitable unrelated donor. Before doing so, a sample of Kate's blood was sent to the Red Cross for specialized and more detailed tissue typing. Now her HLA antigens would be dissected at the gene level to better match with any unrelated person. The results came back five days later, and we entered Kate's HLA typing results in the computer to access the large registry database of the NMDP.

The NMDP was founded in 1988 with the critical involvement of Admiral von Zumwalt, a highly decorated Vietnam War, veteran. He was very active in lobbying Congress to establish such a national registry. He had experienced the importance of a bone marrow stem cell donor firsthand when his son who had been exposed to Agent Orange in Vietnam was diagnosed with lymphoma. Although his son was able to receive a transplant from his sister, Admiral Zumwalt saw many patients who could not find a suitable donor in the family. He realized the importance of a national registry to help those patients.

The NMDP has grown rapidly. In the mid-nineties, only 1.2 million Americans were enrolled as volunteer donors, but by 2010 that number has grown to almost eight million. The NMDP has partnered with registries in other countries whose tissue-typed donors can be searched through a large interconnected database. Almost fifteen million volunteer donors are now available for a patient in need. But the registry is not slowing down, and it continues to organize bone marrow drives all over the country to enroll more donors from ethnic minorities. Instead of blood, only a swab from the inside of the cheek is now needed to determine the tissue type.

In addition to the information about a potential bone marrow donor, an increasing number of *cord blood units* are stored in specialized cord blood banks that can also be searched through the NMDP. These cord blood collections are stored in public cord blood banks. Only a few private or family cord blood banks are available to store and issue cord blood units for an unrelated patient. Cord blood units stored in most of the private banks are meant to be used by family members (Chapter XI.)

Despite the impressive number of over fifteen million bone marrow stem cell donors in the NMDP database, some of the searches are unsuccessful. Chances of finding a donor are better for Caucasians for whom the odds are about 90 percent. Other ethnic and racial groups such as African Americans and Asians still have much lower chances (table 1).

To increase the recruitment of donors from different ethnic backgrounds, the NMDP launched a new Web site (www.bethematch.org) and is also trying to reach the younger generation through social media Web sites. Donors have to be younger than sixty years, must be healthy, and have to pass the same qualifications as blood donor.

As a melting pot, the United States is seeing an increasing number of patients with blood and bone marrow cancer who are of mixed race. For those patients, it is even harder to find a matched bone marrow or cord blood stem cell donor in the registry. Natasha was twenty-six years old when she died of leukemia after a long but futile search for a bone marrow stem cell donor for her. She was of mixed race background and her father was inspired to found the first cord blood bank in the nation with an emphasis on mixed race and minorities (www.natashaslace.org); it operates in conjunction with Cryobanks International (www.Cryo-intl.com), a company that stores the cord blood collections.

Individuals interested in becoming donors should visit the NMDP web site (www.bethematch.org) or attend one of their bone marrow drives. It is easy to become a donor, and no special note on the driver's license is necessary. All that is needed is a swab of the inside of the cheek to determine the individual's tissue (HLA) type. The NMDP will mail a test kit to everybody who is interested in becoming a donor. After the swab is done, it is returned to the NMDP in a preaddressed envelope. A blood test is not necessary initially but might be requested later if a potential donor for a patient is identified.

The need for more volunteer bone marrow donors is also increasing as the baby boomers reach an age where certain blood cancers are more prevalent. As noted earlier, the shrinking family size makes it less likely to find a sibling donor for those patients. Even today, as many as 6,000 patients each year die of blood cancer because no suitable donor for a bone marrow transplant can be found.

Table 1 Volunteer Donors Enrolled in the NMDP Registry by Race and Ethnicity (numbers as of 6/2010)

Caucasian	> 5 million
American Indian/Alaska Native	80,000
Asian	> 450,000
African American	> 515,000
Hispanic or Latino	650,000
Native Hawaiian or Pacific Islander:	9,000
Multiple races	200,000

In order to increase the available stem cell units for transplant, especially for minority groups, Congressman C.W. "Bill" Young, a long-time supporter of bone marrow stem cell transplantation, was instrumental in putting a law in place (Stem Cell Act of 2005) that would aim to increase the number of bone marrow stem cell donors. The act also called for a National Cord Blood Inventory with the goal to collect and store at least 150,000 cord blood units to treat patients. All bone marrow donors and collected cord blood units would be listed in the NMDP database. In addition to the fourteen million bone marrow stem cells donors, it is now possible to also search a network of cord blood banks worldwide. Over 150,000 stored cord blood units are currently searchable through the NMDP database. To become accepted and integrated into the NMDP database, the cord blood banks have to guarantee a certain quality and standard for the collected cord blood units. Private cord blood banks are not part of this network.

Despite this integration, it is still more difficult to identify matched units for ethnic groups other than Caucasians. The private cord blood banks, on the other hand, have over 400,000 units of cord blood stored, an inventory that could provide matches for 90 percent of all patients. However these units were collected and stored under the premise that they would only be used for the child donor or family member, so less rigorous testing was and still is required for those cord blood collections. Hence, the NMDP does not currently include those private banks in the search process.

Kate was lucky; her ethnic background is Caucasian, and she had twelve potential HLA matched donors in the NMDP database. This information can be quickly obtained by performing a preliminary Web–based search of the NMDP database (www.marrow.org).

Now we had to make sure that a repeat and more detailed tissue typing of the donors would match Kate's HLA type. This is the *confirmatory* tissue typing that requires the donor to be contacted for further testing. NMDP was initially asked to test five of the twelve potential donors for Kate. Even if the available tissue-typing information in the database indicated that all twelve potential donors might have been equally good matches based on the tissue type, it is preferred to use donors from the same ethnic background.

Age and the sex of the donor are also taken into consideration. Younger donors are preferred, as the quality of their stem cells is usually better. If possible, patient and donor gender are also matched. A bone marrow stem cell transplant from a female donor given to a male recipient can cause more complications, including rejection and graft versus host disease (GvHD). During pregnancy, women produce immune cells and antibodies in response to the fetus that persist even after the child is born. These immune cells can react with the donor's tissue and can cause more extensive GvHD. A transplant from a male donor to a female patient does not carry the same risks.

All five donors that were identified for Kate had those more favorable characteristics, so the NMDP was asked to obtain confirmatory tissue typing for each. We made sure the NMDP staff knew that this was urgent, as Kate's leukemia seemed to relapse and progress quickly. The NMDP reached out immediately to the five potential donors, but could only contact four of them. It is not uncommon for donors to move and forget to notify the registry. It turned out that one of the remaining four potential donors had recently become pregnant and would not be able to donate. The remaining three individuals seemed to be good candidates, but one of the donors was unable to commit the necessary time required for a stem cell donation because of an upcoming graduate exam.

Two donors remained. Since one of them wasn't as perfect of a match as initially thought, we decided to go with Dirck, a schoolteacher who lived about thirty minutes outside of Amsterdam in the Netherlands.

When he learned that he was tissue compatible with Kate, Dirck was ecstatic at the possibility of helping a patient with leukemia whose only hope was to get a stem cell transplant using his stem cells. He was not allowed to know any details about Kate, except that she had leukemia, was a young mother, and that it was an urgent situation. Kate was also not allowed to know Dirck's name or whereabouts. This is a rule of the NMDP to make sure that patients and their donors don't become emotionally involved. Both are allowed to exchange letters, which are directed through the NMDP office, but they cannot reveal their names. One year after the transplant, their identities can be released, and patient and donor may communicate freely if they wish.

KATE GETS HER STEM CELL TRANSPLANT

Kate was referred to a Web site maintained by the U.S. Department of Health and Human Services (http://bloodcell.transplant.hrsa.gov) that provides in-depth information for patients in need of a transplant, as well as donors. She quite well understood what to expect but had a lot of apprehension. We had to tell her that the chances of dying from the transplant during the first year were about 20 percent and that even the transplant was not a 100 percent guarantee that the leukemia would not come back.

So far Kate had been lucky. Not only did we find her a well-matched stem cell donor, but also it took only six weeks from the initiation of the preliminary donor search until the actual transplant. This time usually is more like eight to twelve weeks and depends on the number of potential donors in the registry and how quickly retesting of the donors can be done. Once the donor has been identified and confirmatory typing has been completed, a physical exam and blood work are also required to make sure that the donor is free of infections such as hepatitis and HIV that could potentially be transmitted with the transplant.

For transplantation, bone marrow stem cells can be obtained in two different ways. The more traditional way is to perform a *bone marrow harvest* under general anesthesia. The procedure is done in the operating room and takes about an hour. The bone marrow is removed from the hipbone through multiple punctures of the bone. Physicians attach a syringe to the needle, and by applying suction, obtain a few milliliters of marrow with each aspiration. This is repeated over and over through the same hole in the skin but at multiple sites in the bone to maximize the stem cell yield. Typically, close to a liter of marrow is removed. This will not affect the donor as the bone marrow cells are replenished from the donor's stem cell pool. However, there is a certain amount of blood loss that goes along with it, and the harvest site may be painful for a couple of days.

More commonly these days, is the collection of bone marrow stem cells from the peripheral blood. To make the bone marrow stem cells come out of the marrow space and into the peripheral blood, the donor is given a stem cell stimulating drug such as Neupogen, which is injected under the skin for several days. The donor is then connected to a machine that is programmed to extract the white cells and return the red cells (erythrocytes) back to the donor.

The machine cannot recognize stem cells and separates cells by size. The collected cell fraction contains mostly leukocytes but also contains the rare stem cell that makes up only about one percent of the white cells. Nowadays more of the bone marrow stem cells are collected from the peripheral blood although bone marrow as a stem cell source still has certain advantages and is still being used. Since the stem cells obtained from the blood originally come from the bone marrow, transplant physicians still call it a bone marrow transplant even if it is actually a blood stem cell transplant.

The transplant center can request either bone marrow or blood stem cells. The choice depends on the patient's clinical situation, age, and disease status. Each source of stem cells has its pro and cons. Stem cells from blood have more lymphocytes, which are highly active immune cells. They may be better to fight any cancer cells left in the patient, but on the other hand, they can cause more graft versus host disease (GvHD) than bone marrow stem cells.

A bone marrow stem cell transplant consists of two main components: depletion and repopulation. First, the patient receives chemotherapy or radiation (or a combination of both), usually at high doses, to eliminate any of the remaining cancer cells in the patient's body. This intensive treatment also causes any healthy bone marrow stem cells to be wiped out, leaving the patient with essentially no functional bone marrow. That's where the transplant comes into play. The second part consists of the intravenous infusion of the donor's bone marrow stem cells. The infused cells migrate to the bone marrow space of the recipient where they begin to regenerate the patient's blood supply, including white blood cells and other cells, such as lymphocytes and natural killer cells that are part of the body's immune system.

Stem cells from blood are preferred in cases where the disease is more aggressive and the additional immune boost can be helpful. Because Kate's leukemia had only stayed in remission for a short period of time, blood stem cells rather than bone marrow stem cells were needed from Dirck. After his blood work showed he had no infections, Dirck received daily injections of Neupogen under his skin for five days. Neupogen stimulates his bone marrow to produce more stem cells and release them from the marrow into his blood.

On the day of the last Neupogen injection, Dirck went to the stem cell collection unit at the hospital in Amsterdam. There he was connected to a machine that passed his blood through a filter to separate and collect the blood forming stem cells. The red cells that were not needed were returned to him through an intravenous needle in his right arm. The entire process took about four hours.

Stem cells have the same size and appearance as many other blood cells, and it is not possible to count under a microscope how many of the stem cells have been collected. The nurse who performed the stem cell collection had to send a small sample of the collected cells to the laboratory to check the number of CD34 cells in the sample. Blood stem cells carry on their surface the CD34 as a marker. Based on the weight of the patient, the transplant center will request the collection of a certain number of CD34 cells. When the result came back from the laboratory, the number was sufficient, and Dirck could be disconnected from the machine. Nothing else would be required from him.

Debbie, the nurse who worked at the transplant center in Amsterdam, picked up the bag containing Dirck's precious stem cells. The cells were placed in a cooler like the type used for camping trips. Debbie then headed to Schiphol Airport in Amsterdam. She had two tickets and the necessary paperwork to allow her to pass through security with the live cells. This was extremely precious cargo. Kate had already received high doses of chemotherapy and radiation. If she did not get the donor's stem cells soon, her chances of dying from bone marrow failure would be close to 100 percent.

Debbie needed the extra plane ticket because the cooler with Dirck's stem cells would be with her all the way placed on the middle seat. Since the temperature of the stem cells must be guaranteed, the cooler cannot be placed in the cargo department of a plane, and the FDA requires that the *chain of custody* is maintained and documented to make sure the collected stem cells arrive in good shape.

On the other side of the ocean, Kate was finishing her countdown for the transplant. She had received three days of radiation to her entire body; the radiation was intended to kill any remaining leukemia cells in her body, and it also weakened her immune system, which was necessary to prevent rejection of Dirck's bone marrow stem cells. Although the cells from Dirck were tissue matched, there remain sufficient differences between them that would lead to rejection if Kate's immune system would not be slowed down by drugs.

In addition to the total body radiation, Kate had received two days of chemotherapy at a very high dose to kill any remaining leukemic stem cells. Another drug, Cyclosporine, was started to prevent rejection and also to prevent GvHD.

Meanwhile, the plane with Dirck's bone marrow stem cells had landed at Logan Airport in Boston. It was almost five o'clock in the afternoon as Debbie passed through immigration and took a taxi to Tufts Medical Center, which is located in the heart of Boston. She knew where she was going because she had delivered bone marrow stem cells there before. Arriving, she went straight to the Blood Bank on the eighth floor and delivered the stem cells to Marcus, the technologist who was waiting for her arrival. He took the precious bag out of the cooler and completed the necessary paperwork.

After Debbie left, Marcus took a small sample from the bag and sent it to the clinical laboratory to have the cells tested for sterility and for the number of CD34 cells. Since the cells had traveled for almost fifteen hours since collection from the donor, it was important to confirm and document that nothing had happened to them. He then labeled the bag, and as soon as he received the clearance from the laboratory, he took the precious cells to the transplant unit where the nurses and Kate were eagerly awaiting their arrival.

Finally it was time. The bag of stem cells arrived, and Kate's nurse hung the cells as if they were nothing more than a blood transfusion. The cells are given through the plastic line that is placed in every patient's arm to make it easier to give infusions and draw blood. After about an hour, the infusion (the transplant) was complete. Kate had no reaction to it. She was surprised how simple the transplant was. Now it would take about ten to fourteen days for her new bone marrow stem cells to settle into the bone marrow space and start producing the new healthy blood cells. It is not clear to physicians and scientists why the hematopoietic stem cells, when given intravenously, know where they have to go and why they settle in the bone marrow space. Research is very active to solve this mystery. Until then we will continue to call this phenomenon "homing" of bone marrow stem cells.

Except for some fatigue, Kate was feeling relatively well the first days after the transplant. But then she began to notice some pain in her mouth. This is a side effect of the chemotherapy that irritates the lining of the mouth and the gut. She had difficulty swallowing and was started on intravenous nutrition to supplement her calorie intake, vitamins, and minerals. Her blood counts by the end of the first week were now all down, and she needed regular blood and platelet transfusions.

At the beginning of the second week after the transplant, Kate developed a fever. This is an expected event after the transplant since Kate's infection fighting white cells were essentially down to zero, and the donor's stem cells had not yet started producing new cells. It was now ten days after Kate's stem cell transplant, and we were expecting some signs of engraftment, which is the time when the new bone marrow starts to function. It remains a mystery to physicians and scientists why there is a blackout period of at least a week before the new stem cells start producing new blood cells. Most likely though, this has to do with the new environment in which the infused stem cells find themselves, and the time they need to adapt.

Kate's engraftment occurred as expected. We noticed that her white cell count had moved from zero to eighty neutrophils (infection fighting white cells) per cubic millimeter twelve days after the stem cell infusion. This was the time when we were watching closely for any signs of graft versus host disease (GvHD). Since Kate's donor was unrelated, we expected some form of GvHD. More often it occurs after an unrelated than after a transplant from a sibling. Unfortunately, physicians have no means of predicting the onset, severity, or the response to therapy. GvHD affects mainly the skin, the gut, and the liver, and its symptoms can be quite uncomfortable. Especially when the gut is involved, diarrhea and cramps can occur. Unfortunately Kate had all three organs involved—and in a major way. It almost killed her.

Kate developed severe diarrhea (several liters a day) and also got a diffuse skin rash that was quite bothersome because of blisters. As soon as the first symptoms developed, we started her on steroids, which are still the best treatment as they slow down an immune response. However, even after higher doses and several days of therapy, her GvHD was still troubling her, and we needed to start another drug that unfortunately did not improve the GvHD. We were running out of options, and I was concerned that Kate would not make it through the transplant.

III.

MESENCHYMAL STEM CELLS TO TREAT KATE'S TRANSPLANT COMPLICATIONS

Dr. Parker, a junior physician in our bone marrow stem cell transplant program, attended the annual meeting of the distinguished American Society of Hematology (ASH) in Orlando, Florida. This conference happens every year in early December and brings together hematologists from all over the world. In one of the scientific sessions, Dr. Parker heard about a clinical trial that had been conducted at the MD Anderson Cancer Center in Houston, Texas, using mesenchymal stem cells (MSC) to treat GvHD. For the trial, MSCs were obtained from young, healthy donors through a bone marrow biopsy and were manufactured and provided by Osiris, a biotechnology company located near Baltimore, Maryland.

The presentation Dr. Parker attended reported that about half of the patients with life-threatening GvHD who were given infusions of MSCs had remarkable improvements. He did not think much about it at the time and was busy keeping up with all the other presentations that were going on at that meeting.

Several days after his return from the conference, Dr. Parker was working in my laboratory again. His project involved the isolation and transplantation (into mice) of MSC from the human umbilical cord, another rich source of MSCs. He mentioned the presentation and the very promising results of MSCs in the treatment of severe GvHD to me in passing. It immediately clicked, and Kate, who was in the intensive care unit fighting for her life with severe acute GvHD, came to my mind. She was having several liters of bloody diarrhea per day, and her kidneys were failing. I immediately 'Googled' Osiris and found their phone number. It was relatively easy to get to the right person at the company.

The medical director at Osiris assured us that they could provide MSCs for our patient, but we had to clear some regulatory hurdles. The FDA had allowed the release of their MSC therapy only under the condition that the ethics board of the hospital approved the treatment on compassionate grounds. Approval for an experimental treatment is usually only granted when patients are gravely ill, and the new and untested treatment is given as a last resort. Such a condition has to be assessed and approved by the hospital's institutional review board (IRB) before the drug, or in this case, the MSCs could be shipped to us.

The next step was to send a summary of Kate's clinical course and a detailed description of her current condition to the IRB at our hospital and ask for emergency approval of the MSC therapy on compassionate grounds. I quickly dictated a summary to the chairman of the IRB and explained in detail why we would need the MSC treatment for Kate. The IRB consists of several physicians from different specialties, a patient advocate, and often a clergyperson. They are not allowed to have any connection to the patient or the company providing the new drug.

After the request for compassionate release was faxed to the chairman of the IRB, we followed up with e-mails and phone calls to make sure that the office was aware that we were working against the clock. Dr. Martin, the chairman of the IRB got back to us within twenty-four hours with a few questions, and then approval was granted. Osiris acted swiftly and sent a team of laboratory technicians to our center. They brought with them a cooler with frozen MSCs. Since our blood bank technicians had never dealt with this type of stem cells, the company's team taught them the process of thawing the cells, how to use the right medium concentration, and how to prepare the right number of cells for infusion.

Things had moved quickly. Kate received the infusion of MSCs only three days after Dr. Parker had mentioned the presentation to me. Everyone—the IRB, Osiris, the blood bank technicians, and our nurses—had come together in a remarkable way. Kate tolerated the first infusion of MSCs without any problems. She was scheduled to get the MSC infusions twice weekly. For the time being she was holding on, although her kidney function had deteriorated to the point where she required dialysis every other day.

It was Friday, and we had given Kate her second infusion of MSCs. So far she was not really any better; however, she had not deteriorated any further. Her blood values were holding, and I was hoping we would be able to buy her some time. The patients who had been treated with MSC infusions at MD Anderson had shown responses after an average of three to four infusions. This made sense as GvHD causes significant tissue damage. Much of the lining in the gut is lost, and in addition to stopping the process, some healing has to occur before one would see clinical improvement.

I was not on call over the weekend, but I phoned the intensive care unit to check how Kate was doing. Her diarrhea had slowed down, and she seemed to have less cramping in her abdomen. Her kidney function was unchanged. When I saw her on Monday, she clearly was much better and had less cramping in her abdomen. This was encouraging and reason for some hope. She received her third MSC infusion on Tuesday, and by Wednesday, it was clear that she was responding. Her stool volume was now less than a liter per day, and her kidney function had improved to a degree that she would need only the occasional dialysis. She was transferred back to our bone marrow transplant unit.

Everybody was stunned because we rarely see a patient with this degree of GvHD take a turn and make it out of the intensive care unit. We continued the MSC infusions twice weekly. Kate was getting better every day and began to eat; at first she could only manage broth, Jell-O, and Popsicles, but she advanced to more solid food. Her diarrhea had almost completely resolved, and her liver-function tests also had significantly improved. Her body rash had turned into a more dry, scaly skin, a clear sign of healing. This was a marvelous recovery, and after being in the intensive care unit with essentially minimal hope, Kate was ready for discharge only three weeks later.

We were also able to reduce the dose of steroids that Kate had been put on to control the GvHD. After discharge, I saw her twice weekly in clinic. Each time she told me that she felt stronger, was eating better, and was slowly getting back to a more normal life. We were able to increase the intervals of her clinic follow-up visits. Her kidney and liver functions had normalized, and her skin had healed completely—clearly a remarkable turnaround considering her dire situation just a few weeks ago.

How did the mesenchymal stem cells (MSC) accomplish such a turnaround for Kate? What are these cells, and why is it possible to give the cells from a totally unrelated individual without problems?

Every organ in our body has its own adult stem cells that can produce new generations of functional, organ-specific cells on demand. These are the adult stem cells. As mentioned earlier, bone marrow is the home to more than one type of adult stem cell: the *hematopoietic stem cell* is programmed to make all types of cells that are circulating in the blood. These are red cells that carry oxygen, white cells (leukocytes) that can fight infections, and platelets that are important for proper blood clotting. It is currently debated and heavily researched whether hematopoietic stem cells have the ability to turn into cells of other tissues such as liver and muscle cells. *Mesenchymal* stem cells (MSC) are the other adult stem cell in the bone marrow, and they have attracted a lot of attention recently. They look like little spindles and make up the supporting structural cells in almost every organ. However, the bone marrow is particularly rich in MSCs. These cells are *multipotential* and can develop across tissue boundaries; they are able to form tissues like bone, fat, cartilage, and even nerve cells. Some investigators have shown that they can tickle them to become muscle and liver cells. It is the MSC that provides structural and nutritional support to the hematopoietic stem cells in the bone marrow space. Beyond that, they behave like little factories that produce chemicals called cytokines, which can stimulate even remote cells in the body.

MSCs have a number of features that make them very attractive for use in humans in the treatment of certain disorders. For reasons not completely understood, they tend to travel to sites in the body where inflammation has cropped up and release some of their cytokines right there to calm down the inflammatory process. MSCs are not recognized by the human immune system and therefore are not rejected by the patient, even if they come from a completely unrelated donor. This means they are universal stem cells that can be obtained from any volunteer donor without concern for tissue (HLA) type, and they can be injected into humans in need for treatment.

The recognition of such universality has prompted the U.S. government to work toward stockpiling a large number of MSCs for emergency situations. What emergency situations could occur remains largely speculation, but most likely the government officials are thinking about nuclear exposure. In 2006 they awarded funding to Osiris to obtain and grow MSCs in large quantities and stockpile them in a frozen state. Osiris had been researching MSCs for a number of years and had developed a proprietary technology to obtain these cells from the bone marrow of healthy donors and grow them in large quantities.

IV.
KATE BECOMES A CHIMERA

A year went by and Kate returned for her anniversary checkup, something that is routine for all transplant patients. In addition to regular blood tests, we look for any signs of *chronic* GvHD, perform a bone marrow biopsy, and assess organ functions. Everything turned out to be fine for Kate, and her bone marrow showed no signs of leukemia. We also examined her bone marrow for the presence of cells from her original donor who was male. This can easily be done by a blood test, checking whether the chromosomes in her new bone marrow were carrying the male Y chromosome. Females have two X chromosomes whereas men have one X and one Y chromosome. In case the donor is he same sex as the recipient, DNA can be analyzed and compared using tests that are familiar from criminal scene investigations.

Before a bone marrow stem cell transplant is performed, the patient is informed that the genetic makeup of his or her bone marrow and blood will change and become that of the donor. The patient will become a *chimera* and will have two different sets of genes in his or her body. In the Greek mythology a chimera was a fire-breathing monster with a lion's head, a goat's body, and the tail of a serpent. When we see female patients for consultation for a bone marrow transplant from a male donor, they sometimes ask if their voice will get deeper. Of course, the answer is no, but some interesting scientific stories have emerged that reveal how *multipotent* these stem cells are. Bone marrow stem cells from the transplant donor can travel through the body of the recipient and settle in various organ tissues.

A group of investigators recently reported that bone marrow stem cells of the donor were found in the finger-nails of transplant recipients many years after the trans-plant. Although scientists don't know exactly what type of bone marrow stem cells are responsible for this effect, it is suspected that the mesenchymal stem cells (MSC) travel to those sites.

Even many years after the transplant, cells from the donor have been found in the heart muscle, brain, and several other organs of the recipient. What effect that has on the patient, if any at all, is currently unknown. But what is amazing is that these cells actually have been integrated into the host tissue and have taken on functions for which they were not initially programmed. As we will see in a later chapter, this can occur because each cell has the full genetic makeup to become any body cell. Certain genes early in the development get silenced but can be unblocked at a later stage.

Chimerism is a fascinating phenomenon. Not surpris-ingly, even Hollywood filmmakers have picked up on it. In an episode of the TV series *CSI*, the DNA from a suspect did not match samples found at the crime scene, though other evidence proved the suspect was the killer. When it was discovered that the suspect had a bone marrow stem cell transplant in the past, and DNA tests confirmed that the samples actually matched the DNA of his donor, the suspect was found guilty.

Researchers at Yale University recently discovered male donor cells in the lining of the uterus (the endometrium) of women who had received a transplant from male donors. This is remarkable in so far as endometrium cells are shed every few weeks during menstruation. This means that stem cells from the donor's bone marrow became embedded into the endometrial lining. They must be long lived and contribute to the renewal of the endometrium cell cycle. Although it originally was a bone marrow stem cell, it now can make different cells. Researchers call this *plasticity*. At this point, scientists have to admit that they don't quite know how this can happen.

In addition to fingernails and the uterus, bone marrow stem cells from the donor have also been found in hair follicles of patients who had received a bone marrow stem cell transplant. The observation by scientists at Duke University that transplanted donor cells can localize to the heart of a bone marrow transplant recipient has triggered a number of clinical studies in patients with heart problems. In these studies, bone marrow cells are given directly into the coronary arteries or even directly into the heart with the hope and intention of improving heart function after a heart attack.

Scientists at the Fred Hutchinson Cancer Research Center in Seattle have found that cells from the human bone marrow can settle in the brain of the transplant recipient. When the researchers looked at brain tissue of female patients that had died of transplant-related complications, they saw male donor nerve cells in their brain tissue. This was a surprising finding: how did they get there and how did they turn into nerve cells – we don't have the answers..... yet.

Certain allergies to food or pollen or even asthma can also be transferred from the donor. This happens because memory-immune cells are transferred with the donor's bone marrow and settle in the patient's bone marrow.

And then there are the stories for which we have no explanation. A female patient who had received a bone marrow transplant from her brother became almost addictively interested in watching and reading about all kind of sports, although she had not been interested at all in sports before the transplant. When she opened a newspaper, she turned first to the sports section. Even when watching TV, she was flipping channels just to find a sports game. Although her brother, the stem cell donor, had an interest in sports, he did not have the same "craving", as she called it. Is it possible that the bone marrow stem cells in the brain of our recipients were responsible for some *rewiring*? This remains a mystery for now.

After the transplant, the patient's bone marrow stem cells are replaced by those of the donor. The new stem cells also produce the cells that now make up the patient's immune system. Immune lymphocytes, which can detect even small differences between tissues, recognize the donor's cells as foreign and launch an attack. During this time, the new immune system is essentially in overdrive, not only attacking the patient's healthy cells (and causing graft versus host disease) but also cancer cells that may be left after the chemotherapy.

For decades, physicians and scientists had argued about whether the immune system can control the growth of cancer cells. This question was not decided until the *graft versus cancer* effect was discovered in patients after a bone marrow transplant. When a twin is the donor for the patient, the graft versus cancer effect will not occur because there are not enough differences between them to stimulate the donor's immune cells. Interestingly, for that reason, the relapse rate of the blood or bone marrow cancer after a twin transplant is much higher.

Fortunately, Kate's leukemia stayed in remission, and as of her last follow-up appointment, she is now leukemia free for more than five years. Most relapses after a bone marrow stem cell transplant occur within the first two years, and we would consider Kate cured of her disease after that point. Kate was very grateful for having been given this extra time because she was able to see her son graduate from high school and finish college.

When we transplanted Kate, we had to use high doses of chemotherapy and total body radiation to kill all possible leukemia cells in her body. Her disease was bouncing back quickly, telling us that we needed heavy weapons to keep the disease from recurring. In many patients with less aggressive disease, we will get by with less intense chemotherapy and radiation. In some cases, the transplant treatment is so well tolerated that it can be performed on an outpatient basis. These types of transplants are also known as *mini-transplants*. The reduced intensity of the transplant regimen for mini-transplants also allows older patients (in some cases up to the age of seventy-five) to undergo this treatment.

V.
CANCER STEM CELLS: THE BAD ACTORS

I recently attended a cancer conference and was late for a presentation about cancer stem cells. When I walked into the conference room, I saw a slide that showed dandelions and a lawn mower, and I wondered if I was at the right conference or was the speaker up to something interesting? It turned out that he was talking about the dandelion theory of cancer treatment.

Here is how it goes: the cancerous transformation makes some cancer cells like a stem cell and they are able to replicate themselves and more importantly they can put out hordes of more mature cancer cells. A cancer stem cell like any other stem cell, can maintain itself through self-renewal. The cancer stem cell is like the queen bee, producing offspring that are uniform cancer cells whose growth is limitless.

When physicians look at the blood of leukemia patients, they see leukemia blasts all over and after chemotherapy, these blasts disappear, but the leukemia stem cells will not necessarily be affected by the treatment and disappear. The leukemic stem cells can be resistant to the chemotherapy and survive. What does this have to do with dandelions? Chemotherapy works like a lawnmower—it cuts the top of the dandelions (the cancer blast cells), and the lawn looks pretty and nice but often only for a limited time. Since the lawnmower left the roots behind, the dandelions can grow back and at some point they may spread over the entire lawn and mowing will only give temporary relief. Unless better drugs are developed that actually get rid of the roots of the dandelions (the cancer stem cells), chemotherapy alone will not always cure cancer. The exception is when chemotherapy can be combined with a stem cell transplant; in this case not only are healthy stem cells transplanted, but also a new immune system is given to the patient that can keep the leukemia stem cells (dandelions) in check.

Drug companies are eagerly working to learn more about cancer stem cells in order to develop more specific and more effective cancer drugs. This still remains a challenge because in many diseases it is difficult to pinpoint the cancer stem cell and to target it such that normal healthy cells are not affected.

VI.
STEM CELLS TRANSPLANTS FOR AIDS?

Infection with the HIV virus can cause AIDS, which makes the person prone to all kinds of infections. Today's drug treatment for HIV positive persons (called HAART) can prevent progression of the disease and if taken early enough and consistently, patients may not even develop full-blown AIDS. Despite this effective treatment, the patients' immune system still may not be completely normal, and patients at a later stage can develop lymphoma or leukemia as a consequence of the immune deficiency.

The activity of HIV infection can be measured by the number of cells called CD4 lymphocytes in the blood. These lymphocytes are the ones that get attacked by the HIV virus, get infected, and inactivated. Those CD4 cells however are also at a crucial juncture for the activation of the patient's immune system to help it fight infections and recognize cancer cells. In these days methods are available to measure the actual HIV load even at low levels in a patient using sensitive techniques. If the CD4 count is normal (over 200 cells/ml), and the viral load is low, it usually predicts a better prognosis. Although the HAART drug treatment has been very effective in controlling the disease, the medication has to be taken without interruption, at times has unexpected side effects, is expensive and not always covered by an insurance plan.

In 2008 an American living in Berlin (Germany) who was infected with HIV, developed acute leukemia. He needed a bone marrow stem cell transplant but had no tissue-matched siblings that could be his stem cell donor. Being Caucasian, he had a good number of tissue-matched potential donors in the NMDP registry. The physicians at the Charite Hospital in Berlin went one step further in the donor selection and did special tests on those potential donors to find out if any of them had a mutation for the gene that codes for the cell surface protein CCR5. In order for the HIV virus to enter a lymphocyte, it uses two different receptors (hooks) on the human lymphocyte: the CD4 and the CCR5. If CCR5 is blocked or is not present, then the HIV virus cannot enter the lymphocyte and destroy the patient's immune function.

The patient's physicians were able to find a stem cell donor for him who was well tissue matched and most importantly, lacked CCR5 - a lucky coincidence since only one to three percent of the population carries this genetic mutation.

In preparation for the transplant, the patient was given high doses of chemotherapy to kill off his own bone marrow stem cells and any residual leukemia cells. The bone marrow stem cells from the donor took in a timely manner after the transplant. Since the immune lymphocytes were now generated by the transplanted healthy bone marrow stem cells, the newly produced CD4 lymphocytes could not get infected because they were not carrying the CCR5 receptor for the HIV virus. It has been more than two years since the transplant, and the patient has not required any HIV drugs, and no virus can be found in his blood. The number of CD4 cells is in the normal range, and he is free of infections.

A bone marrow stem cells transplant for this man was performed because he had leukemia. Those transplants are not done and should not be done to treat AIDS. Current HAART medication is quite effective in keeping the disease under control. However, there is a growing population of AIDS patients that lives much longer than before, which has increased the chances of developing a bone marrow or blood cancer. Some of those patients can benefit from a bone marrow stem cell transplant. In those cases it can be useful to screen for a donor who lacks the expression of the CCR5 molecule on the surface of his or her lymphocytes. Since only 1-3 percent of the population carries this genetic defect, most transplant candidates will not have an available donor with this particular genetic variant.

This story however is important from another perspective: is there another way of obtaining stem cells that carry the CCR5 deficiency than relying on a particular bone marrow donor? Can bone marrow stem cells be altered such that their CCR5 gene is inactivated?

A number of new technologies have become available to silence or inactivate genes of interest. These technologies have fancy names like *antisense technology* and *RNA interference*. Unfortunately these technologies work only temporarily as they don't change the genetic makeup of the stem cell permanently. To accomplish a more permanent change *gene scissors* may be the future. This new technology has been used successfully in fruit flies to cut out a particular gene and is also widely used in agriculture to generate genetically engineered plants and crops. But this sounds easier than it technically is. So far it has been mostly trial and error. The challenges are to get those molecular scissors into the right place to make them work at the right spot of the complicated gene.

Even if research succeeds in successfully converting a few stem cells, those would have to be expanded to large numbers to support a patient and to be able to reconstitute a new bone marrow functionally. So far, expanding the bone marrow stem cell has been challenging. However there is encouraging news from the Fred Hutchinson Cancer Research Center in Seattle, where scientists were able to engineer a protein that can be used to activate a certain pathway in stem cells and make them multiply and expand more than hundredfold.

VII.
DIAGNOSIS MYELOMA: USING PATIENT'S OWN BONE MARROW STEM CELLS

Larry was a sixty-one-year-old recently retired airline pilot. He had been feeling well and according to his recent annual checkup had just received a clean bill of health. One summer weekend, he was mowing his lawn, when he tripped over the mower's power cord. It wasn't a major incident; he just fell to the ground and used his left arm to break his fall. He experienced a sudden sharp pain in his arm and heard a clicking noise that immediately told him that he'd broken his arm. An x-ray confirmed that he indeed had fractured his left arm. This was unexpected because his fall wasn't especially hard.

His physician suggested getting some additional x-rays of other bones and run some additional blood tests. He also needed surgery to stabilize his arm. The test results unfortunately were not good. They showed that he had a high level of an abnormal protein in his blood. The presence of this *paraprotein* is typical for *myeloma*; it is caused by cancerous growth of a certain cell type of cells (plasma cells) in the bone marrow that produce the abnormal protein. Importantly the x-rays of his spine showed that he had some additional bone "defects" there as well which could be troublesome and cause compression of his spinal cord if not treated properly.

Myeloma is a hideous disease that over the years has become more prevalent and aggressive and is also affecting more and even younger patients. The increased concentration of the paraprotein in the blood can affect organ function, particularly kidney function. The cancer cells also produce other chemicals, and while most of them have not been fully elucidated, it is known that they can eat away the bone, make it brittle, and can cause fractures that occur unexpectedly, without a substantial impact, just as Larry experienced.

Larry needed treatment, and his physician started a combination of two drugs. One was steroids, and the other one a new drug that interferes with the life cycle of plasma cells. The majority of patients responds quite well to this therapy and can stay in remission for several months, but ultimately the disease will come back. Despite the progress in the treatment for myeloma that has been accomplished by new drug combinations, relapse and crippling complications are the norm. The only treatment that has shown to get rid of the disease is a bone marrow stem cell transplant from a sibling or matched unrelated donor. However many older patients don't qualify for this treatment, and many physicians will therefore advise they have an *autologous* transplant first.

An *autologous* transplant uses the patient's own bone marrow stem cells collected before high doses of chemotherapy, to protect and rescue the patient from the effects of the chemotherapy. The bone marrow stem cells for an autologous transplant are generally obtained from the blood before chemotherapy. In preparation for the stem cell collection, the patient receives one day of chemotherapy, which is followed by daily injections of a blood-stimulating hormone (such as Neupogen or Mozobil). This combination will push the bone marrow stem cells from the marrow into the blood. This process is called *stem cell mobilization*.

Two weeks after the initial round of chemotherapy, Larry came back to have his stem cells collected and frozen. He had a needle placed in his arm and was hooked to a machine that is programmed to filter out the white blood cells—thereby also capturing the stem cells—and then returning the red cells back to Larry's blood. The process usually takes two to four hours and, except for the needle stick, is not painful. The collected stem cells are then frozen and stored in liquid nitrogen at a temperature of minus 320° F. A special cryoprotectant is added to make sure the stem cells remain viable while in a frozen state.

After the stem cell collection, Larry was given a couple of weeks off to recover before he started the actual transplant sequence. Most transplant centers nowadays perform at least part of the autologous transplant sequence for myeloma patients in an outpatient setting. During the treatment, the patient can stay either in special housing on the medical campus or even at home if the driving distance is within certain limits.

Larry lived a twenty-minute drive from the Medical Center, was a reliable patient and his wife and teenage children were very motivated to look after him. We told him that he would have to come to clinic every day to have his blood counts checked and his kidney and liver function tested.

About two weeks after we had Larry's stem cells collected, he came back to the clinic to receive high-dose chemotherapy, which consisted of a single infusion of the chemotherapy drug Melphalan. He was also given drugs to prevent nausea and vomiting. After a couple of hours everything was over, and Larry could go home.

He returned the next day for the stem cell infusion. Two technicians from the blood bank had brought the frozen bags with his stem cells to the clinic. The stem cells would be thawed and then immediately infused because they can lose some of their activity when they are exposed to the cryoprotectant too long after being thawed.

The stem cells, suspended in a saline solution, were given by intravenous infusion; Larry was immediately aware that he was receiving the infusion because the cryoprotectant (DSMO) gives the patient a certain taste. Every patient will speak of a different taste—fish, garlic, or metal. Staff and visitors also notice a smell for the first day after the infusion, typical of a patient who has received an autologous stem cell transplant. Larry tolerated the infusion well and just felt a bit "squeezy" in his stomach. After a couple of hours, he was ready to go home with the appropriate instructions.

Larry's daily visits went well. His white cell count (leukocytes) dropped to very low levels as expected and three days after the stem cell infusion, he told us that his mouth felt sore, which is a common side effect of the melphalan chemotherapy. In some patients the mucositis becomes more severe, and they have a hard time swallowing despite pain medication. If the mucositis becomes more of a problem, painkillers and intravenous nutrition to supplement the decreased calorie intake may be necessary.

It was the fifth day after the stem cell transplant. Larry's blood leukocytes had been very low for the last couple of days. When he came to clinic, he reported about feeling quite fatigued, and he had a fever of 101.8° F. Despite being on prophylactic antibiotics at home, he had caught an infection.

Larry needed antibiotics and intravenous fluids, and we decided to admit him to the inpatient unit. He recovered quickly on intravenous antibiotics, and after having been without fever for twenty-four hours, he was sent home. He was now eight days after the stem cell infusion, and we expected him to recover his blood counts over the next few days. Patients usually know quite well when their bone marrow function is starting to recover. Even when the white cells are still very low, they usually tell us that their mouth is less painful. They also feel their physical strength coming back. Larry had an unremarkable course and was able to return to his daily activities after a few weeks.

We continued to see him in our outpatient clinic on a weekly basis, and after a couple of months, we transferred his care back to his oncologist closer to his home. As of his last follow-up appointment, which was two years after the autologous transplant, he is doing well and enjoying an early retirement.

VIII.
A CORD BLOOD STEM CELL TRANSPLANT FOR ROHIT

Rohit, a financial consultant with a large firm who lives in Bermuda, just got married; he turned thirty-four years old just a few weeks ago, and he and his wife were planning to start a family. Rohit was looking into getting life insurance to secure his and his family's future.

Before issuing the policy, the insurance company required that Rohit get a physical exam and some basic blood tests. He was feeling well, had absolutely no health issues and had no reason to believe anything unexpected would come up. Unfortunately it did. He received a phone call from the insurance company who told him that some more blood tests were needed before they could issue the policy and that he needed to see a hematologist. The white cell (leukocyte) count in his blood was slightly higher than normal. The usual range is between 4,000-8,000 cells per mm^3 blood volume, but in his case, the number was 18.000. All the other numbers in his blood were normal.

The next day Rohit asked his primary-care physician for a referral to a hematologist, and on Monday, he saw Dr. Matthew for what he thought would be a quick visit. He had Googled high white blood count and had found that the most frequent cause was an infection that caused an outpouring of young cells that could be seen on the blood smear. So he was not really concerned about the high number of white blood cells.

When Dr. Matthew saw Rohit in clinic, he noticed that his spleen was somewhat enlarged. The nurse took some blood and told him it would be sent for a special test called FISH (fluorescence in situ hybridization). This test can identify chromosomes in the blood cells that can be "painted" with a specific fluorescence dye. Abnormal chromosomes will light up. The results of Rohit's FISH test showed that a short piece of his chromosome 9 had been broken off and relocated to chromosome number 22.

Since chromosomes contain the DNA, the blueprint and code for all the proteins our body makes, Rohit's bone marrow stem cells were now making an abnormal protein called *bcr/abl*. It causes the cells in the bone marrow to divide and multiply much faster; many more cells, especially young cells, are sent out into the blood. This abnormality of the chromosomes is typical for chronic myeloid leukemia or CML for short. The new chromosome that is formed by the translocation between the two ends is known as the *Philadelphia chromosome* as it was first discovered and described in a patient from Philadelphia.

Chronic myeloid leukemia (CML) can affect patients of all ages, and its course is hideous. It may go on for some time without causing any problems or being detected. Rohit's story of getting the diagnosis incidentally during an insurance exam is not unusual. Although we don't know exactly what causes the chromosomes to break and join another one, it is interesting to note that survivors of the Hiroshima atom bomb explosion have developed CML at a much higher rate than the normal population.

Compared to just a few years ago, treatment options for CML have changed dramatically. Until then the only treatment that could be offered was a bone marrow stem cells transplant from a donor to replace the diseased stem cells. Although such a stem cell transplant provides a cure for the majority of patients, it still carries a certain failure risk, and one of ten patients will die during the first year. The only drug available in the past to control CML cells was Hydrea, which just keeps the elevated white cell count under control but does not change the course of the disease.

 Then along came a new class of drugs, so revolutionary they made the cover of TIME magazine. The "wonder drug" is Gleevec, and it was the first drug of a new generation of drugs of *small molecules* or *targeted therapies*. Gleevec snaps on to the bcr/abl protein made by the aberrant Philadelphia chromosome and neutralizes its deleterious effects on the cells.

Clinical trials would confirm that the majority of patients taking Gleevec would achieve a normal leukocyte count and a few would get rid of the Philadelphia chromosome altogether. However, when investigators were starting to look more closely at the gene level of the cells, they could still find the bcr/abl abnormality in most patients. Some hematologists were skeptical that Gleevec would just keep a lid on the disease and would not get rid of the malignant clone (the "bad" stem cell). In addition, the drug had some side effects, and some of which were more serious such as fluid retention in the lungs and around the heart. Some patients also developed resistance to Gleevec treatment. Meanwhile second and third generations of Gleevec-like drugs have been developed, and they provide some hope for those who have become resistant to Gleevec.

ROHIT'S CML DOES NOT RESPOND TO TREATMENT

Cancer stem cells are smart. They are capable of adapting to changing conditions and can escape the effects of drugs. Hematologists also are starting to learn more about the leukemic stem cell that can lie quiescent for some time while not dividing, which means that Gleevec and similar drugs cannot attack them as effectively since those drugs only target actively dividing cells. Despite the skepticism, Gleevec and other *small molecule drugs* undoubtedly have their benefit by delaying the transformation of the disease to a more aggressive stage. They do not however remove the leukemic stem cell that can only be accomplished by a stem cell transplant.

Rohit unfortunately did not respond to Gleevec and also experienced some of its side effects such as fluid retention in his legs. We therefore decided to start him on the second generation of small molecule drugs for CML that works much like Gleevec. However, the chances of a response are drastically diminished once a patient's CML has become resistant to Gleevec. We told Rohit that we needed to look for a stem cell donor for him and to be ready for a transplant. The writing was on the wall.

Rohit had no siblings. When we searched the database of the National Marrow Donor Program (NMDP) for an unrelated stem cell donor, we quickly noticed that it would be very difficult to find a match for him in the registry because of his ethnic background - Rohit was from Sri Lanka. Unfortunately, even a search for a closely matched cord blood unit turned out to be negative.

Rohit had read a lot about his disease, its treatment options, its outcome, and about a stem cell transplant. The average time for a CML to turn into an acute leukemia (blast phase) is about three to five years, and we did not know how long Rohit had his disease before it was diagnosed.

During this time in Boston, away from his family who remained in Bermuda, Rohit stayed in an apartment close to the Medical Center that he had rented. It was January and Boston was experiencing a harsh winter. Understandably, Rohit had a hard time being in Boston by himself during those winter days. One night during a phone conversation with his wife, she told him that she was pregnant, and he couldn't have been happier in those moments. But after his joy had settled, some more rational thoughts came to his mind: what if his CML didn't respond to the new drugs and no stem cell donor could be found for him. Should he bank his child's cord blood—could they be used for him?

There was still a chance that a matched cord blood stem cell unit for Rohit would come up in the national database, as the NMDP was making substantial efforts to increase the number of cord blood units, especially from ethnic minorities. But Rohit knew he could not rely on it. By having his baby's cord blood cells frozen away, he thought he would at least have a potential donor from the family. When he came to clinic the next day, he had a lot of questions, and we talked about cord blood transplantation in more detail.

When a baby is attached to his or her mother in the womb, blood flows from the baby through the umbilical cord to the mother's placenta where it is recharged with oxygen and nutrients. Early in the pregnancy, the baby makes blood cells in the spleen or in the liver. The bone marrow takes over only in the last few months of the pregnancy. After delivery, when the baby's cord is clamped, some of the baby's blood is trapped in the placenta and the umbilical cord vessels, and can be extracted by the obstetrician with a syringe.

The blood from the placenta and the cord is rich in adult stem cells and particularly hematopoietic stem cells that can be used for a transplant. These stem cells are much more potent than stem cells obtained from the bone marrow and hence less numbers are needed than from an adult person. In addition, the stem cells are "younger" and have a longer lifespan ahead of them. The drawback is that the immune system of the baby has not been exposed to any infectious diseases and has not developed any solid immune response that could protect the transplant patient.

In addition, the stem cells in cord blood take longer to take, to produce new blood cells, and the patient is left without sufficient numbers of infection-fighting leukocytes for some time. But there is an advantage of using cord blood over bone marrow or blood as a source of stem cells for transplant—because the immune cells in cord blood are less mature, the recipient and the patient don't have to be perfectly matched with one another.

Since the first cord blood transplant on a boy in Paris in 1988, over 15,000 cord blood stem cell transplants have been performed worldwide, mainly in patients with blood or lymph node cancers. In 2005 the U.S. Congress passed the Stem Cell Research and Therapeutic Act, to create a National Cord Blood Inventory of at least 150,000 high-quality cord blood units stored in public cord-blood banks. The Institute of Medicine, which advises Congress, arrived at this number, which according to its calculations would have enough donor units available from for all ethnic backgrounds to provide to patients in need of a transplant.

Umbilical cord blood from volunteer donors is frozen and stored in public cord-blood banks, in contrast to private or family cord-blood banks (chapter XI), that store the baby's cord blood cells for use only by relatives. However, if the baby's cord blood cells are donated to a public bank, the source would remain anonymous, and the donated cord blood cells could not be claimed by the mother or the child in the future. Since Rohit was thinking of storing his child's cord blood cells with the idea of possibly using it for his own transplant, his cells would have to be stored in a private cord blood bank.

Rohit had heard that for many adults, the number of cord blood cells that can be obtained from a baby's cord, often have insufficient numbers of stem cells to support a transplant for an adult. The minimum cell number that is required for a cord blood transplant depends somewhat on how well the patient and the cord blood donor are tissue (HLA) matched. Unfortunately only 10 to 20 percent of all adult transplant candidates will have enough cells in a single cord blood unit available to safely undergo a transplant. The story is slightly different for children in whom a compatible unit with enough stem cells can be found in over 90 percent of all cases.

To overcome this shortcoming, some transplant centers will pool two cord blood units from two different babies. This seems to work to a certain extent, but it also increases the costs of a transplant. Cord blood banks usually charge about $35,000 for providing a cord blood unit.

Another way of getting around the low number of stem cells in cord blood is to expand their number using special devices called *bioreactors* that provide oxygen and nutrients and some growth hormones to the cord blood stem cells. After a couple of weeks in a bioreactor, the cell number has increased. Although this sounds very elegant and straightforward, the technology is not quite there yet but biotech companies are eagerly working on it.

A big advantage of using cord blood stem cells for transplant is that the stem cells are available right away like a blood transfusion. No donor work up is necessary and there is no inconvenience for the stem cell donor.

Time went by and Rohit's CML was reasonably stable, but his bone marrow still had the Philadelphia chromosome suggesting that his disease could progress anytime. His wife's due date was approaching and both came to Boston for the delivery. Rohit had put everything in place, so that his baby's cord blood cells could be stored with one of the private cord blood banks in the Boston area. He was aware that the chances that his baby's tissue (HLA) type was reasonably closely matched were remote, but he felt that this was better than having no stem cells available. So it came as no surprise to him when the results from the tissue typing came back and his son was only half matched and was not the first choice for a transplant.

After his return to Bermuda, Rohit's CML seemed to cause more problems for him. He was developing some anemia, a decline in the red cells that carry the oxygen in the blood. A bone marrow biopsy confirmed concerns that his disease had progressed. Time was running out. Fortunately we had kept the unrelated stem cell donor search for Rohit open. The government's intense efforts to increase the number of unrelated donors especially in the cord blood registry seem to have worked in his favor: two closely tissue matched cord blood units with a sufficient stem cell number had now come up in the database. They were better matched and had a higher number of stem cells than the one that were stored from his child.

The two cord blood units for Rohit were stored in different blood banks—one was in Australia and the other in Belgium. Fortunately our transplant coordinator could submit all the paperwork through the National Marrow Donor Program (NMDP). The cord blood units had to be at our hospital before Rohit could begin the preparative chemotherapy regimen. The chemotherapy and the radiation are high dose, and Rohit's bone-marrow function would not recover without the transplanted cord blood stem cells. So we had to make sure the stem cells actually made it from the two different continents safely. Cord blood cells are shipped in a cryoshipper, which is essentially a thermos that keeps the cells in a frozen state. At the bottom of the cryoshipper is a little computer chip that records the temperature to make sure it is kept at a safe level during the long travel hours.

Our hospital had to purchase the two cord blood units at a cost of $70,000 total. They were delivered to our blood bank that kept them frozen until the day of the transplant. Upon arrival, a small blood sample was obtained to confirm that the cord blood units were indeed the correct ones.

After Rohit had received three days of chemotherapy and three days of radiation, it was time for the cord blood stem cell infusion. The bags with the cord blood cells were taken from the freezer, thawed, and brought to the transplant unit. The cord blood stem cells were given through his intravenous line and the "transplant" was over in less than half an hour.

As expected, it took about four weeks for Rohit's new stem cells to start working and produce blood cells. The reason for the delay is that the cord cells are quite immature and need some time to get acclimated to the new bone marrow environment. Rohit had a number of expected complications such as infections, some kidney problems, and some mild GvHD, but we could discharge him some six weeks after he was admitted. He stayed close to the medical center in an apartment that the hospital provides, and we continued to see him regularly in our clinic. After three months, he was able to go back to Bermuda. We stayed in close contact by e-mail and phone with him and his physician on the island. When he came back for his checkup one year later, he looked very well, his CML was not detectable, and his ordeal was almost forgotten.

IX.

A TREASURE FOR ADULT STEM CELLS: BONE MARROW AND UMBILICAL CORD BLOOD

Bone marrow stem cell transplants have been performed for the past fifty years, initially only for patients with end-stage leukemia who had exhausted all their treatment options. The success in these advanced-stage patients was rather modest. Still, a small percentage of those patients survived and became long-term survivors. Those early transplants were performed at the Fred Hutchinson Cancer Research Center in Seattle, that initially tested the concept of bone marrow transplants in dogs who had developed lymphoma. In the years to come, transplants were done for patients whose leukemia could be pushed back into remission, which resulted in more than half of all patients surviving for many years. The Seattle transplant team was headed by Dr. E.D. Thomas who received a Nobel Prize in 1990 for his pioneering work in bone marrow stem cell transplant.

Now, bone marrow and cord blood are increasingly recognized as a potent source of multipotent stem cells that can do things beyond just replacing a cancerous stem cell in the bone marrow as we saw for Kate, Larry, and Rohit. Scientists and physicians working in different disciplines are discovering their tremendous potential, and we are just learning what those and other adult stem cells and embry-onic stem cells may be able to do for patients tomorrow.

At this point, we know that there are at least two differ-ent types of adult multipotent stem cells in bone marrow and in cord blood (figure 2): hematopoietic stem cells *(HSC)* and mesenchymal stem cells *(MSC)*. To replace their leukemia stem cells, Kate had received new hematopoi-etic stem cells from the blood of an unrelated person and Rohit had received cord blood. The transplant provided both with healthy hematopoietic stem cells that could produce new blood cells for them - those essential cells that fight infection, carry oxygen, and can stop a bleed.

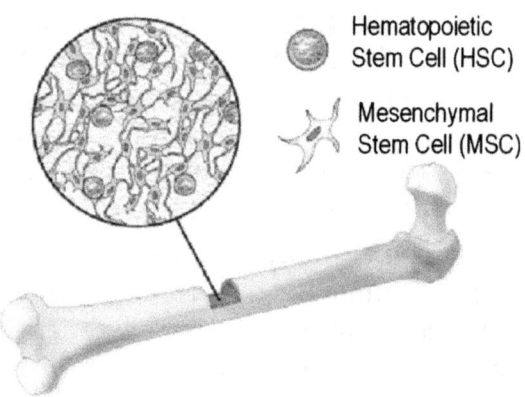

Hematopoietic
Stem Cell (HSC)

Mesenchymal
Stem Cell (MSC)

Figure 2

Inside of our bones is marrow that is the site for the hematopoietic stem cells (HSC) responsible for the production of blood cells. The HSC are found in close proximity to the mesenchymal stem cells (MSC), which provide structure and nutrition to HSC. Mesenchymal stem cells are multipotent and can be coaxed into becoming carti-lage, bone, muscle, fat, and nerve cells.

Beyond the hematopoietic stem cell, bone marrow and umbilical cord blood harbor a second type of multipotent stem cells—mesenchymal stem cells (MSC). When Kate developed severe GvHD after the transplant, she received a preparation of MSC that slowed down this overshooting immune reaction and in the end saved her life. In addition to controlling the overshooting immune response of GvHD, MSC also produced unique proteins that helped heal Kate's organs after the transplant.

In the bone marrow, MSC not only provide support structure for the hematopoietc stem cells but also some "nutrition," essentially maintaining the well-being of those precious hematopoietc stem cells.

The supportive role of MSC for the hematopoietic stem cells was first discovered when scientists made an observation in mice that were specifically bred to accept human stem cells and not reject them. One of the unresolved problems after a cord blood transplant is the delayed return of bone marrow function (engraftment), especially the production of white cells (leukocytes). However, when the scientists transplanted human cord blood cells and also infused mesenchymal stem cells (MSC) into mice at the same time, they noticed a more robust and faster engraftment of the cord blood cells.

The MSC can come from any donor and don't have to be tissue matched. They are not rejected by the recipient, which is surprising to many scientists but makes MSC universal stem cells. Another advantage of MSC is that they can be prepared in large quantities and stored frozen, which makes them easily available.

It is quite likely that both bone marrow and umbilical cord blood contain additional types of adult multipotent stem cells that are not yet known and characterized but could be of therapeutic use in the future. Scientists suspect that bone marrow and cord blood contain endothelial or vascular stem cells that are capable of forming new small blood vessels.

Mesenchymal stem cells (MSC) tend to home in on sites of inflammation and may even target cancer sites. They have a "homing device" that sends them to the point of injury in the human body. For that reason they are also explored as vehicles for anticancer drugs that can be released locally. This research is at an early stage but potentially represents an interesting way to reduce the side effects and toxicity of systemic administration of chemotherapy that can cause so much collateral damage to normal cells.

Some biotech companies are taking the MSC from the bone marrow and exposing them to some stimulants to generate a more specialized, more differentiated mesenchymal stem cell (MSC) before they are administered to the patient. One way is to expose MSC to a specific nerve growth factor to push the development of MSCs in the direction of nerve cells. Those more dedicated cells could be more effective in treating brain disorders such as Parkinson's or Alzheimer's diseases. At this point, only studies in rats have been done and trials in humans are pending, and at least five to seven years away.

BONE MARROW STEM CELLS FOR ARTHRITIS, MENISCUS AND BONE REPAIR

When MSC from bone marrow are placed in a plastic dish, they can be coaxed into cartilage, bone cells, connective tissue, and even muscle and nerve cells. With these abilities, MSC are the prime candidates to revolutionize *regenerative medicine* that will help to repair damaged tissues and organs. In fact some tissue cells (muscle, bone and cartilage) are relatively easy to generate from MSC. However, to get a three-dimensional tissue structure that resembles an organ, it takes the involvement and input from engineers to design the right scaffolds that tell the cells how to form and align. It also needs bioreactors to grow the cells with exactly the level and composition of nutrients found during natural cartilage or bone development. This is still a formidable challenge, but research in this area continues to be very active. Here are some examples.

With our aging population, the number of individuals with arthritis is reaching epidemic proportions. Since MSC from bone marrow can turn into cartilage and bone cells, they have become the center of research for this condition. Unlike bone, cartilage does not grow back. Damaged cartilage in arthritis can lead to joint pain and loss of physical function

Osiris, the biotech company that has specialized in research and production of human mesenchymal stem cells (MSC), tested their product in goats whose joints were affected by arthritis. When MSC were injected into the joints of these animals, healing of the cartilage surface was observed within a couple of weeks (figure 3). A clinical trial in the United States is ongoing at several medical centers to find out whether injection of MSC into the knee of patients whose arthritis has become painful, can improve symptoms.

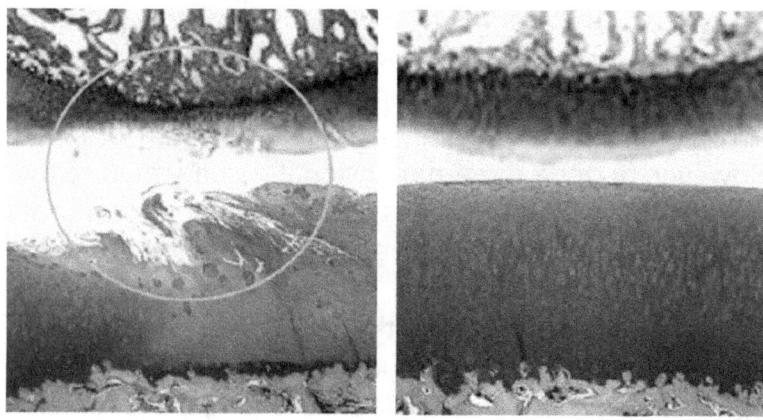

Figure 3

In arthritis, the surface of the joint has become uneven and rough due to cartilage erosion (left). On the right side the same joint is shown several weeks after MSC had been injected into the joint. The MSC contribute to cartilage formation, but they can also release certain chemicals that can help to rebuild the cartilage surface (picture courtesy of Osiris Therapeutics Inc.)

Injuries and degenerative changes of the meniscus are common in our aging and exercise-oriented society. The most common treatment in case of meniscus injury is to surgically remove it; this leaves the leg bones in the joint without any cartilage "cushion." A recent study tested whether the injection of mesenchymal stem cells (MSC) into the joint would improve symptoms after the affected meniscus had been removed. This was a blind study, and half of the participants did not get the MSC injections. At assessment one year later, the individuals who had received the MSC, had significantly less symptoms and pain.

Mesenchymal stem cells (MSC) from bone marrow are finding their place in tissue engineering. For example, Preparations of MSC are used by surgeons to promote healing of bone fractures or to fill in bone defects after injury.

Scientists and engineers at Columbia University in New York recently created a jawbone, part of the joint used for chewing, for a patient using her own bone marrow cells as a starting material. Aside from stiffness and pain, the jawbone can be destroyed by disease, injury or birth defects. The team initially used digital images from the patient's jaw to design an appropriate mold. The cells were then cultured using a special bioreactor that was designed, so that it would infuse the growing tissue into a mold.

The engineers demonstrated with this important work that they could engineer a piece of bone with the right dimensions - which is critical when it comes to repair of bone defects. The next step in this direction will be to engineer a bone graft that will also include cartilage - a first step toward replacement of an entire joint engineered from the patient's own bone marrow mesenchymal stem cells (MSC). Future studies will also have to show that the bone is strong enough to withstand compression and torsion.

Other exciting developments have been reported using mesenchymal stem cells (MSC) from bone marrow. Doctors in Spain recently build a new trachea (windpipe) from bone marrow cells. A young woman had previously suffered from tuberculosis, which had caused some scarring in her lungs leading to a narrowing of her trachea . She had significant breathing difficulties and couldn't even adequately care for her two children or function on a day-to-day basis.

To rebuild the windpipe (trachea), the physicians first removed the windpipe from a diseased person and treated it with chemicals that removed any remaining tissue except the cartilage rings that supports the windpipe. They then harvested bone marrow cells from the woman's hip and grew them up in culture. Once the scientists had enough cells, they coated the trachea scaffold with those bone marrow-derived mesenchymal stem cells (MSC). Some cells from the airway lining were added also. After a few days to allow the cells to grow into the scaffold, the windpipe was inserted into the lung bronchus of the patient. The implant is working well, and the patient's condition has improved remarkably.

Mesenchymal stem cells are part of several biomaterials that can be placed on wounds to promote faster healing. The cells are also part of the extracellular matrix (ECM) that represents a gemisch of proteins, molecules, collagen fibers, and MSC. Extracellular matrix can be found in every organ, and its function is to provide structural support to the surrounding organ tissue. Extracellular matrix has been in the news lately. The Pentagon has pushed research on ECM as it promises to rebuild muscles of legs and hands after injuries. ECM is extracted from the tissue of pigs, and it can be processed in powder form.

Because ECM is obtained from pigs, soldiers have nicknamed it "pixie dust." ECM have recently be shown to help regrow some muscle tissue. In order to do so, ECM are placed on a scaffold that is then applied to the wound area (www.cbsnews.com/stories/2009/12/11/60minutes/main5968057.shtml?tag=contentMain;contentBody). The pixie dust powder itself doesn't regrow the missing muscle; it tricks the patient's body into doing it itself. More recent studies suggest that bone marrow stem cells circulating in the blood use the ECM as a guide to morph into new muscle cells and that the environment in the tissue tells the bone marrow stem cells which cell type they have to become.

BONE MARROW STEM CELLS FOR HEART DISEASE

There are different heart conditions for which stem cell treatments are currently tested (i) angina, where patients have reduced blood flow to certain areas of the heart resulting in intermittent chest pain that at times can be significant, (ii) heart attack, which is the result of an acute blockage of the coronary artery resulting in the death of tissue in certain areas in the heart and (iii) heart failure as a consequence of chronic low blood circulation and consequently, low oxygen to the heart muscle, which leads to weakened pump function. Heart failure also occurs when cardiac muscle is damaged after a heart attack and scar tissue replaces beating heart cells. As scar tissue replaces healthy tissue, it causes the heart to enlarge and lose its pumping capacity. This can cause the heart to fill with fluid, which moves to the lungs and can lead to all kinds of organ complication. To assess the pump function of the heart, doctors use the left-ventricular ejection fraction (LVEF) as a yardstick.

A search on www.clincialtrials.gov will list many active trials across the country that are recruiting patients for different types of stem cell treatment protocols to cure those heart ailments. For most trials the patient undergoes an aspiration of bone marrow from the hip. The cells are then separated from the red cells and given intravenously to the patient. Alternatively, the bone marrow stem cells are injected directly into the blocked artery. Most centers will administer the separated leukocytes from the bone marrow with no further processing since the multipotent stem cells will be included. It is not resolved a this point which route of injection of bone marrow stem cells is the best.

Since bone marrow contains both hematopoietic stem cells and mesenchymal stem cells (MSC), it remains speculative which stem cell type contributes to a beneficial effect. A clinical trial performed at the University of Miami did show that the intravenous infusion of purified bone-marrow-derived MSC could improve heart function. Those MSC were off the shelf MSC obtained from young healthy volunteer donors. The patients who received MSC had an improved pump function of the heart and also had fewer irregularities in their heartbeats

Stem cell therapies are also explored for chronic heart failure. Some biotech companies take the patient's MSC obtained from his or her own bone marrow and use a cocktail of cytokines to turn them into heart-like cells. They claim that these cells will be better suited to regenerate damaged heart muscle than MSC that have not been further manipulated.

If the coronary artery is not completely blocked, but the blood flow is just intermittently impaired, patients can experience chest pains (angina), which at times can reach a debilitating level. A recent study, performed at twenty-five medical centers across the nation, reported that patients receiving stem cells from their bone marrow experienced less pain and were able to better exercise without pain. Physicians used a sophisticated mapping technology to determine the specific areas of the heart that were alive but not functioning properly because of reduced oxygen delivery to those areas. They then injected the bone marrow stem cells directly into the site hoping that those stem cells would stimulate new vessel formation.

Since this study was not controlled against a group of patients that were treated exactly the same way but received only an injection of normal saline (placebo), it is impossible to say if this treatment really had any benefit. Some patients may have experienced subjective improvement - simply the fact that they had received a cutting-edge medical treatment made them feel better.

At this point, it is difficult to say if any type of stem cell treatment for heart conditions brings about more than a marginal benefit. Are stem cells really needed? Researchers at the University of Buffalo using an animal model reported that heart function could also be improved when bone marrow cells were injected into a leg muscle or even when an extract of bone marrow cells was given to the animal. This suggests that any beneficial effect may potentially be due to some chemicals they produce and that direct contact may not entirely be necessary.

There is a lot of enthusiasm among cardiologists about stem cell therapy for the heart, but the truth is, we don't know if it really benefits patients and if it does, how it works. A lot of questions remain unanswered but stem cell therapies are a hot area and any reputable heart center likes to have this treatment included in its portfolio of services offered.

BONE MARROW STEM CELLS TO IMPROVE LIMB CIRCULATION

Bone marrow stem cells can either differentiate into, or induce and augment the growth of new, small arteries. It has been shown in animal studies and in some early clinical trials that the injection of the patient's own bone marrow stem cells into the skin and the muscle of the limb can improve the blood flow through formation of new small vessels. Improved circulation and healing of ulcers, even in diabetic patients, was observed.

Patients also reported that their walking distance had improved after the procedure, which had a positive effect on their quality of life. What is needed now are controlled clinical trials that consist of a patient group that is not given stem cells but just saline injections (placebo) to make sure these improvements are real and not just based on the psychological effect of a medical procedure. One also needs to know whether this treatment in the end will avoid otherwise necessary amputations.

BONE MARROW STEM CELLS FOR PREMATURE BABIES?

Babies who are born prematurely often do not have fully developed lungs and need to be hooked up to mechanical respirators and oxygen machines to help them breath. Unfortunately, the machines can also damage the babies' fragile lungs by forcing oxygen into them, stretching the tissue, and causing micro bruises. This complication can be deadly or, if the baby survives, can leave it with chronic lung disease. For example, babies born at twenty-four-weeks gestation - sixteen-weeks premature - have an 80 percent chance of developing chronic lung disease compared to 50 percent of babies born at 28 weeks.

Researchers in Canada injected bone marrow stem cells directly into the lungs of prematurely born rats with lung problems and observed that the rats had much better healing and recovery. To their surprise, however, they could not find the bone marrow cells in the lung tissue, and it is quite possible that the injected cells just released some chemicals that were responsible for the healing process. Although these observations are exciting, it will take probably two to three years before trials in babies will be underway.

Patients in the intensive care unit are often placed on a respirator to support their breathing. Sometimes lung injury from the mechanical ventilation develops which makes it almost impossible to wean the patient off the machine. Researchers induced a similar lung damage in rabbits and reported that the intravenous injection of bone marrow cells markedly improved their lung function, reduced the water in the lungs, and decreased bleeding. Most likely this is mediated by the mesenchymal stem cells (MSC) in the bone marrow. Clinical trials should follow soon.

BONE MARROW STEM CELLS FOR SPINAL CORD INJURY

This devastating condition leaves many individuals disabled forever and bound to a wheelchair. In addition to cord blood cells and possibly embryonic stem cells (Chapter XIII), a patient's own (autologous) bone marrow cells are being studied for treatment. In a clinical trial in Korea thirty-five patients with complete spinal cord injury had their bone marrow cells injected into the surrounding area of the spinal cord injury site. A control group of patients was treated with conventional standard treatment.

Although about one-third of patients had some minor improvement, approximately 20 percent of the patients who got the bone marrow injection reported increased pain around the injection site and the paralyzed body parts. These results were somewhat disappointing especially since studies in rodents had a much better outcome. However there are important differences between the rodent and the human spinal cord and any of the new stem cell treatments will have to be tested in nonhuman primates.

UMBILICAL CORD BLOOD STEM CELLS

Some exciting breakthroughs are reported with umbilical cord blood stem cells. These treatments go beyond of just replacing a bone marrow that has been affected by leukemia as in Rohit's case. We are learning that cord blood contains several different types of multipotential stem cells, the building blocks for bones, heart, liver, and the nervous system. Some scientists believe that cord blood may even contain pluripotent stem cells that are more closely related to embryonic stem cells. The truth is that scientists have not yet characterized all the stem cells that may be in cord blood and really don't yet know their full potential.

Umbilical cord blood stem cells are free of any political and ethical debate. In fact, many states are introducing legislation to mandate education of pregnant women about the option of storing their baby's cord blood. Storage can be arranged with a public or private cord blood bank (Chapter XI).

Scientists at Duke University have shown that cord blood cells can actually turn into heart muscle cells and produce an enzyme that is typical for heart muscle cells. The way they found out about this phenomenon was quite serendipitous. A four-year-old boy who had received a cord blood stem cell transplant for a congenital metabolic disorder, died of complications. On autopsy donor cells were found in the heart of the boy. What the doctors don't know yet is whether the cord blood cells of the donor had transformed into heart muscle cells or whether they had fused and combined with them.

The following are some additional examples of recent discoveries with umbilical cord blood cells, some of which have already led to treatment of patients.

CORD BLOOD STEM CELLS TO MAKE BLOOD FOR TRANSFUSION

There is a great need for blood transfusion and the supply of sufficient numbers of units strictly depends on blood donors. Not surprisingly there are situations when hospitals struggle to find blood with the matching blood group to transfuse patients. This supply issue is particularly prevalent in the battlefield where wounded soldiers may need large numbers of transfusions. Blood transfusions also carry a certain risk of transfusion reactions and transmission of diseases. Although donor screening in our country is very comprehensive, there are always emerging pathogens that carry the risk (albeit remote) to be transmitted.

Although biotech companies have worked on developing artificial blood, this has largely been unsuccessful. In order to address the increasing demand especially in the battlefield, the Department of Defense has made funds available to develop technologies that would churn out blood group O blood that can be given to any recipient without blood group matching. This initiative is paying off and some biotech companies are reporting that they can get up to 20 blood units for transfusion, generated from a single cord blood collection. At this point work is ongoing to lower the production costs. If successful transfusions from cord blood generated blood stem cells could become a reality soon.

CORD BLOOD STEM CELLS TO BUILD HEART VALVES

Doctors in Germany have built new heart valves from umbilical cord blood stem cells. They thawed frozen umbilical cord blood cells and seeded them on a biodegradable scaffold of heart valves that they then grew in the laboratory. Current replacement heart valves are made from porcine material, or they are metal (steel). If those heart valves are implanted, the patient has to take blood thinners lifelong to prevent the formation of blood clots on their surface. Clots can be dangerous when some part of the material breaks off. Those microclots can travel to the brain and cause strokes.

Heart valves grown from patient's cord blood stem cells do not have this problem and wouldn't require blood thinners. Another benefit of these cord blood derived heart valves is that they could last throughout the patient's lifetime because they are not rejected and change shape as needed. Children who have received an artificial heart valve outgrow them as they grow older and frequently need repeated heart surgery to replace the outgrown valve.

CORD BLOOD STEM CELLS FOR DISORDERS OF THE BRAIN AND NERVES

Cord blood cells are currently tested in animal models to see if they can slow down the process of degenerative diseases of the brain. These diseases are common in older patients and are becoming more prevalent as our populations ages: Alzheimer's, Huntington's, Parkinson, and Lou Gering's disease. Abnormal proteins that accumulate in the brain and lead to functional brain defects are a common element of each of these diseases—that is about all we know about them. Unfortunately there are no new, more effective therapies available that would slow down the progression and the mental decline.

The effect of cord blood stem cells on these diseases has not been tested in humans. There is some evidence from studies in rats that injection of cord blood cells improved their brain function: the animals were induced to develop Parkinson's disease and then had cord blood stem cells injected into their brain. Compared to a nontreated control group of animals, treated rats had delayed symptom onset and progression of Parkinson, as well as prolonged survival. It is not entirely understood how this improvement is happening. A similar phenomenon can be seen in aging rats. When they received cord blood cells, the age-related decline of brain function could be delayed. Cord blood cells have also shown to improve the physical and behavioral deficits of animals after an experimentally induced stroke. Although these experiments in animals appear to be promising, one has to keep in mind that behavioral changes in rodents may be more difficult to assess and may not always allow for the simple conclusion that this may also work in humans.

Physicians at the University of Texas at Houston are studying whether infusions from cord blood stem cells stored at birth, can improve outcome in children with traumatic brain injury. The same group of physician researchers has already shown that bone marrow, obtained from the child's pelvis, processed and then infused into his or her blood can bring about some recovery after a brain injury. In the absence of a control group, the question is how much the children would have improved without the infusion of bone marrow stem cells.

Muscular Dystrophy is a hereditary disease of the muscle whose cells lack a certain essential enzyme called dystrophin. Children with this disease have a progressive decline of the skeletal muscles and hence muscle strength. The disease only affects boys who can become confined to a wheelchair at young age and end up on a breathing machine because their own breathing muscles are no longer working. Cord blood stem cells can differentiate into muscle cells and when put in contact with muscle cells affected by muscular dystrophy, can induce some regeneration of muscle tissue. As for so many other stem cell treatments, this has only been shown in animals with studies in humans pending.

Can cord blood stem cells some day be used to improve our hearing as we age? It may seem possible, although so far it has only been shown in mice that this actually could work. Mice were made deaf by exposure to a drug known to cause inner ear damage and a high intensity noise. Those mice had human cord blood cells injected into their blood and the researchers were surprised to find the cord blood cells in the inner ear of the animals. When they compared them with a group of deaf mice that had not received any cord blood cells, they found that structures of the inner ear had been repaired and behavioral analysis suggested that some hearing had been restored.

CORD BLOOD STEM CELLS FOR CEREBRAL PALSY

Cerebral Palsy is one of those devastating brain disorders that develop early in a child's life as consequence of a number of circumstances that have affected the developing brain during or shortly after birth or even during infancy. It can affect body movement, posture, and muscle coordination, as well as learning, hearing, vision, and cognitive skills. Risk factors for cerebral palsy include premature birth (under thirty-seven-week pregnancy), prolonged oxygen loss during delivery, or infection and other incidents during the pregnancy or during the first years of life of the child. A recent report by the March of Dimes estimated that one out of every ten pregnancies in the United States results in premature delivery with an increased risk of developing neurological problems in early childhood.

So far, more than fifty children with cerebral palsy have received infusions of their own stored cord blood stem cells. Although it may be difficult to attribute any beneficial effect solely to the cord blood infusions, some success stories have been reported: (www.msnbc.msn.com/id/23572206/) and (www.channelnewsasia.com/stories/singaporelocalnews/print/1022138/1/.html)

Clinical trials are urgently needed to determine the real impact of cord blood stem cells in this disorder. Tuscon Medical Center and the Cord Blood Registry (www.cordblood.com), a commercial stem cell bank, have recently teamed up to store umbilical cord blood from newborns thought to be at risk for developing cerebral palsy. The program is called Newborn Possibilities, and the cord blood will be stored for five years free of charge. A similar trial is now also underway at Duke University (www. pediatrics.duke.edu)

CORD BLOOD STEM CELLS FOR SPINAL CORD INJURY

No real progress has been made in the treatment of traumatic spinal cord injuries. Although there are a number of encouraging observations in animal models, very few patients have received stem cell treatments. A report from China described four patients who were given an injection of cord blood cells. As with other reports that involve only a few patients treated, it is difficult to say if the slight improvement that was reported, was truly due to the cord blood stem cells. This is not a procedure without risks, especially if cord blood cells from an unrelated person are used. There could be a local reaction that could make symptoms worse and cause some pain sensation, as it has been observed with the injection of bone marrow cells in another study.

Instead of cord blood stem cells, embryonic stem cell injections are just entering clinical trial and will be discussed in a later chapter (XIII).

CORD BLOOD STEM CELLS FOR DIABETES

Diabetes can strike in early adulthood (also called type I diabetes) and results from a destruction of those cells in the pancreas that produce insulin (islet cells). Insulin controls the blood sugar level. The attack on the pancreas cells is caused by the patient's immune system that for a yet unknown reason turns against its own tissue. Patients become dependent on insulin injections for the rest of their life. Insufficiently controlled blood sugar levels over time can cause organ damage and patients with diabetes are at higher risk for heart disease, renal failure, and vascular complications such as blindness and stroke.

In the laboratory it has been shown that cord blood cells can be coaxed into insulin-producing cells. The hope is that these cells can be transferred to the patient and would start producing insulin. Unfortunately this has not yet been successful. If a patient's own cord blood cells are available, this would at least get around the problem of rejection.

Researchers at the University of Florida are taking a slightly different approach. By infusing a patient's own stored cord blood stem cells, they are testing whether children can obtain better blood sugar control without being so dependent on insulin. Since cord blood also contains mesenchymal stem cells (MSC), which are known to dampen an immune response, cord blood may contain any self-destructive process by the patient's own immune system against the insulin producing cells. However this may only work at the very beginning of the disease before the islet cells have been destroyed.

CORD BLOOD STEM CELLS FOR CONGENITAL METABOLIC DISORDERS

The stem cells transplant team at Duke University has performed cord blood transplants for congenital metabolic diseases in young children. These hereditary disorders are characterized by the absence of specific enzymes that the body needs to break down and get rid of byproducts of energy production. These byproducts can then accumulate in organs and influence their function, which can be particularly bad when the developing brain is affected. The scientists at Duke have shown that cord blood stem cells migrate to the brain and can provide some replacement for the missing enzymes.

Children with these rare metabolic diseases regained organ function more rapidly when they received a transplant of cord blood stem cells rather than conventional bone marrow stem cell. Since these metabolic disorders affect organ function over time, it is important that the cord blood stem cells are transplanted early before potentially irreversible organ damage has developed, even when the baby is still in the womb. In this case the cord blood cells are injected directly into the baby's abdomen at three to four months into the pregnancy. For this form of treatment, the cord blood cells are usually obtained from a public cord blood bank and come from an unrelated donor. Since the baby's immune system is not yet fully developed at such an early stage, the infused cells are not rejected.

X.
STEM CELLS FROM OTHER BODY PARTS

Each tissue in the body carries adult stem cells that are usually just *unipotent* and are responsible for supplying functional cells for the organ they are residing. It has long been known to physicians that damaged or burned skin can be replaced by healthy skin taken from a different body area of the patient. These skin transplants are possible because of the presence of unipotent stem cells in the bottom layer of the skin. Now scientists learning to grow new skin from small pieces of the skin that are put in culture dishes and stimulated to grow.

Another example for the use of unipotent stem cells comes from England. Physicians there recently treated patients with adult stem cells to restore their eyesight. Those patients had injuries to their cornea, which is the membrane that covers the front of the eye. If this protective layer is not present or damaged, every blink is painful and the eye is prone to infections. The stem cells that generate and maintain the cornea cells can be found in a pocket at the outer border of the eye. Patients had their stem cells taken from that area, grown up in the laboratory and then transplanted onto the eye. Vision in all patients improved and their pain eased.

An example for *multipotent* stem cells comes from a site one would not readily suspect—the upper part of the passageway in our nose carries the olfactory stem cells. Olfactory cells are responsible for our sense of smell. If stimulated in the plastic dish with a cocktail of chemicals, they can form nerve cells (neurons) more readily than cells from any other place in the adult nervous system. This area of the nose can be accessed quite easily and scientists believe that the olfactory stem cells are particularly suited in the treatment of neurological diseases, stroke, or spinal cord injuries.

In Portugal, patients with severe spinal cord injury who were unable to use their legs had those olfactory cells injected into their spinal cord. Surgeons also removed some scar tissue from that area, and afterward the patients underwent an intense rehabilitation program. Remarkably, some patients were able to walk with assistance and walkers. It is difficult to say though how much the transplanted olfactory stem cell contributed to this improvement. The surgery and the intensive rehabilitation may have had provided some benefit of their own. Regardless, these observations are encouraging and physicians and researchers in the United States are now conducting a similar trial in the United States.

Another stem cell source for regeneration of nerve cells is the brain of the fetus. Functionally committed cells can be obtained from the brain tissue of aborted fetuses (sixteen- to twenty-gestational week). These cells have been injected into the brain of mice that had a congenital enzyme deficiency that is also seen in humans. The transplanted fetal cells engrafted and started producing the missing enzyme. The same cells have also been used in rats to treat age-related macular degeneration of the eye, which affects older people and impairs vision over time. The biotechnology company that conducted the studies in rats claims that the animals had better eyesight after the treatment. Studies in humans are on the drawing board.

Some clinics and hospitals abroad inject brain cells from aborted fetuses into the brain of children with brain disorders. These treatments are very problematic as they are done in a less regulated environment in which not even the quality of the cells is guaranteed. A recent report from Russia, where a boy had received brain cells from an aborted fetus had an unexpected outcome—the boy developed brain cancer that originated from the injected fetal brain cells (www.isscr.org/public/briefings/danger.html)

A British biotech company is about to begin a safety trial in the United Kingdom for disabled stroke patients. Nerve stem cells are directly injected into the affected area of the brain. The nerve stem cells are obtained from a cell line that has been obtained in 2003 from brain stem cells of an aborted fetus. The company had tried to get permission from the FDA to conduct the trial in the United States, but the agency had problems with putting cells from a human fetus into the brain of a patient who essentially does not have a fatal condition.

Most organs of our body carry mesenchymal stem cells (MSC) that provide structural support to the particular organ. As we saw before, these MSC are multipotent stem cells equipped to convert into bone, cartilage, muscle, and even nerve cells. The hallmark of MSC is that they can convert into various cell types, depending on the stimulating medium they are put in when they are cultured.

Research is discovering that there are certain tissues from which even more versatile MSC can be obtained. These tissues include the placenta, the amnion fluid (which surrounds the fetus in the womb), and the umbilical cord itself. Many of these organs are discarded after delivery, but an increasing number of stem cell banking companies are offering to isolate and store these potentially useful cells.

In order to understand the differences between MSC from different organs and their potential to regenerate tissue, we need to take a closer look at the tail end of the chromosomes that carry our genes. Each of our chromosomes (and we have forty-six in each cell) carries specific DNA gene sequences that sit like a baseball cap on their ends. They are called *telomers* (figure 4). The function of the telomers is to give some stability to the chromosomes and also protect them from any external influence that would make them fragile.

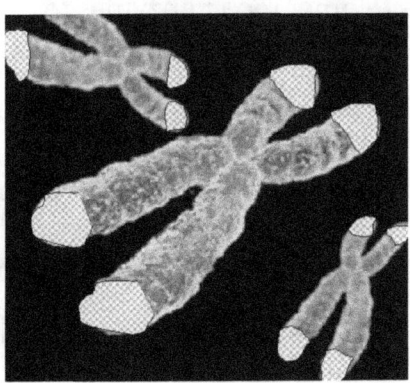

Figure 4

A cluster of three chromosomes that carry our genes. At each of their ends they have telomers, little caps of coiled DNA that protects them from getting shorter.

Each time our cells divide, the telomers get a bit shorter. Although human cells carry a repair enzyme for the telomers that eagerly works on rebuilding the telomers to full length, it can't keep up with the loss of the telomers over time. The shortening of telomers essentially reflects the aging process of our cells. It is believed that if science discovers how to maintain and elongate the telomers, we could delay the aging process. With the shortening of the telomers, the genes also get more exposed to cancerous mutations.

In cancer cells, the repair enzymes for telomers are very active and essentially prevent the cancer cells from dying. Some researchers speculate that manipulating (i.e., blocking) those repair enzymes in cancer cells could force their natural death which could lead to new drugs for cancer treatment. Research on aging on the other hand is trying to activate the telomer repair enzymes to extend the lifespan of healthy body cells and potentially delay their aging.

There are some inherited disorders in which the repair enzymes don't work well. Patients with these congenital diseases age prematurely. A young kid can look like an old person with all the degenerative diseases such as skin wrinkles, heart disease, and arthritis manifested at an early age.

What do telomers have to do with mesenchymal stem cells (MSC) from different tissues? The umbilical cord and the placenta are especially rich sources of early, more primitive MSC that have longer telomers and will have a longer lifespan ahead of them. In addition these stem cells have not been exposed to external events that would change their genetic makeup and are relatively pristine. Hence these stem cell sources are an ideal starting material for stem cell therapies.

In addition to having longer telomers, MSC from fetal tissues also carry certain genes that are closely related to those of embryonic stem cells. These genes have fancy names like Nanog, Oct4, and Sox. When these genes are activated, the cells can revert back to a state like an embryonic cell and when appropriately "tickled," can transform into cells of different tissue quite similar to what embryonic stem cells can do. Scientists are currently using these genes and introducing them into all sorts of cells to make them more like embryonic stem cells (chapter XIII). The generated cells are called iPS, which is short for induced pluripotent stem cells. In the future it may be possible to selectively activate these genes if they are dormant in a cell by stimulating them with certain chemicals and growth hormones. MSC from fetal tissue, in addition to being pristine, are easily accessible and represent an ideal starting cell source for generating iPS cells.

STEM CELLS FROM THE UMBILICAL CORD

The umbilical cord is rich in early mesenchymal stem cells (MSC). The cord is about two feet long and carries two arteries and a vein for the blood flow between the baby and the placenta on the mother's side (figure 5). These vessels are embedded in a viscous pliable material that was first described by the English physician Dr. Thomas Wharton (1614-1673). This Wharton's jelly can easily be extracted from the cord and grown in large quantities.

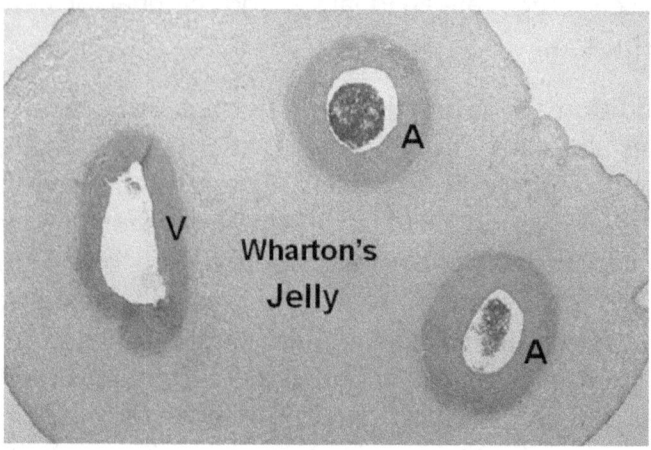

Figure 5

Cut through an umbilical cord. In addition to two arteries (A) and one vein (V), the umbilical cord is made up of Wharton's jelly, which provides protection of the large vessels. The Wharton's jelly is a rich source of mesenchymal stem cells (MSC).

After the baby's delivery, the umbilical cord is discarded. It is now increasingly recognized that the Wharton's jelly cells represent an easily accessible, non confrontational source of early MSC. Just by freezing a piece of cord, these cells can be preserved forever.

MSC are not rejected when infused into an unrelated person, not even when given to another species. This makes it possible to test human MSC in experiments with rodents and monkeys. When cord MSC were injected close to the brain lesion after a bleed or stroke, they significantly improved brain function in rats. Researchers believe MSC from umbilical cord prevented a damaging inflammatory process in the stroke area of the brain and promoted new vessel formation. Other research has found that jelly cells injected into the brain of rats that were induced to develop Parkinson disease, resulted in improvement in their behavior compared to a control group that did not get the cells.

Some private (family) cord blood banks have begun to offer banking jelly cells from the cord especially in combination with the collection and storage of cord blood cells. Future parents now can elect to save a piece of the baby's cord at the same time the cord blood is collected by sending both to the private cord blood bank in prearranged kits. Public cord blood banks have not yet implemented such a simultaneous storage.

STEM CELLS FROM THE PLACENTA AND AMNION

Cells from the placenta are also rich in early mesenchymal stem cells (MSC). While cord blood and the umbilical cord (containing jelly cells) can be collected relatively easily by a health care provider at the hospital, the placenta must be sent to a specialized laboratory for processing before the stem cells can be recovered. As such, placenta stem cell collection and processing is more labor intensive than umbilical cord stem cell processing, and so far, very few private banking companies offer this service.

While the fetus is in the womb, it is floating in a little balloon, a sac that carries the amniotic fluid. The fluid protects the growing fetus. The membrane that constitutes the amniotic sac is the *amnion*. Both the amniotic fluid and the amnion contain early stem cells. With regard to their potency, these cells are considered somewhere between embryonic and adult stem cells.

STEM CELLS FROM FAT

Fat cells (called *adipocytes*) are embedded into the structural mesh of mesenchymal stem cells (MSC). After removal of the fat cells, the MSC can be teased into becoming cartilage, bone, or muscle cells. It is intuitive to think that MSC from fat tissue can easily be obtained in high cell numbers. Biotechnology companies making the point that the cells are ideal for aesthetic body contouring and plastic surgery, such as breast reconstruction.

Engineers came up with a small device that washes the harvested fat tissue and drains the tumescent fluid, fat, and any tissue debris in less than half an hour. This allows the patient's own fat tissue to rapidly be prepared for re-injection back into the same patient. More research needs to be done to find out if the MSC from fat tissue have the same abilities as MSC from bone marrow, from the cord and the placenta.

The use of MSC from fat cells is already in place in veterinary medicine. Racehorses who suffer a ruptured Achilles tendon or meniscus lesion are treated with their own fat MSC. For this procedure, veterinarians will remove fat cells (usually from the back of the horse). It is then sent to a laboratory that will separate the MSC from the fat cells, grow them in culture, and return them to the local veterinarian who will inject them into the joint to stimulate new cartilage formation or support the healing of a tendon.

STEM CELLS FROM TEETH

Recently teeth have been discovered to contain adult stem cells. Both baby teeth and adult teeth contain small numbers of multipotent adult stem cells (so called pulpa stem cells) but also some MSC like cells. Both can be found inside the tooth close to its bottom and center.

Although pulpa stem cells can produce some components of teeth (pulp and dentin), it is still unclear if they can be used to obtain all the other essential parts that are needed to build a tooth. Recently a group from Italy though used dental pulp stem cells to rebuild the crest of a jawbone in a patient to better anchor the teeth.

Dental pulp cells are genetically more closely related to nerve cells of the brain, and some scientists believe that those cells at some point may be better suited than stem cells from bone marrow for the treatment of brain disorders such as Parkinson disease and stroke. Researchers at Emory University's Yerkes National Primate Research Center in Atlanta implanted dental pulp cells from rhesus monkeys into the brain of mice. The dental pulp cells stimulated the growth of nerve cells and some of the injected cells actually turned into brain cells.

Dental stem cell banking companies are springing up (www.ndpl.net). They charge between $500 and $1,500 for the initial tooth preparation and about $100 annually for storage. A collection kit with the appropriate medium can be obtained from the company. The tooth just has to be dropped into the vial, and the box mailed back to the bank. As with other stem cell banking, the consumer takes a risk whether those cells will ever be used.

STEM CELLS FROM MENSTRUAL BLOOD

Recently it was discovered that menstrual blood, as it is shed from the lining of the uterus (called endometrium), contains adult stem cells. These stem cells, termed endometrial regenerative cells (ERC), can be collected relatively easily during the menstrual period. The banking company will send a special collection 'cup' to the client that is returned to the company for cryostorage.

Although the endometrial regenerative cells (ERC) look like and have a lot in common with mesenchymal stem cells (MSC) from other organs, the company claims that there are some differences and scientists believe that they have some preference to differentiate into particular tissues. Like with other stem cell sources, it remains to be seen if the initial observations in the test tube and in animal models can be reproduced in humans.

STEM CELLS FROM HUMAN BLOOD

If menstrual blood contains adult stem cells, than one should assume that blood that gushes through our body also contains those valuable cells. After all, hematologists use stem cells from blood to transplant patients with leukemia. Unfortunately it is not that straightforward. The number of both the hematopoietic (HSC) and the mesenchymal stem cells (MSC) is low and it requires enrichment methods to get to meaningful numbers. The hematopoietic stem cells can be released from bone marrow by injecting a blood stem cell stimulating drug (i.e. Neupogen) for a few days, which can drive those stem cells from the bone marrow into the blood.

Some companies have sprung up claiming it is useful to freeze blood stem cells in case they are needed at a later point in life to support a transplant for leukemia or any other blood and lymph node cancer. The collection is quite expensive—in the range of $10,000—and quite inconvenient. The client has to inject the blood stem cell stimulating hormone for a few days before being connected to a stem cell collection machine. Although the procedure is relatively safe, side effects like bone pain related to the injection of the stem cell stimulating drug frequently occur.

Stem cell collections from blood as an insurance policy for treatment of cancer at an undefined point in the future should not be recommended. Leukemia is better treated with bone marrow stem cells from a sibling or unrelated donor to capture the immune benefit of the donor cells. Most lymphoma patients don't have bone marrow involvement and the blood stem cells can be obtained at the time when a transplant is being considered, so prophylactic storage is unnecessary. And what are the chances anyway for an individual to develop lymphoma and needing a stem cell transplant?

Even if the consideration is to use those blood stem cells for regenerative medicine, other stem cell sources like the bone marrow and fat will be much easier to access and to obtain when actually needed.

XI.
STEM CELL BANKING

Of about five million births in the United States each year, more than 99 percent of the cord blood stem cells are discarded as medical waste. Currently, less than a half of the states in the United States require that expectant parents receive information from their obstetrician about their options to bank their baby's cord blood in public or private banks. Hopefully this number will grow. In 2005 the *Institute of Medicine* recommended to the U.S. Department of Health and Human Services the establishment of a national policy for the banking and use of lifesaving stem cells derived from donated umbilical cord blood (www.bloodcell.transplant.hrsa.gov).

The Institute also recommended that an organization be put in place that would manage daily operations of public cord blood banking and allocation nationwide. The idea behind this recommendation was to assure that more hematopoietic stem cells for transplanting patients with leukemia and other blood cancers would become available especially for certain ethnic groups that are not well represented in the national bone marrow registry. Although it is possible to match for the HLA tissue type between patient and donor, patients do better if they get stem cells from a donor with the same ethnic background.

Carol was expecting her first child, and she faced difficult decisions concerning her child's cord blood. Should she bank her child's cord blood, and if she decided to do so, should she donate it to a public bank or store it for her child's or family's use in a private cord blood bank. She was confused about which route to pursue, or if she should even bother to bank the cord blood. She had read that the private banks required an upfront processing fee and an annual storage fee for the cord blood.

Public cord blood banking is free, but since it is an anonymous donation, it is no longer possible to use the cord blood stem cells for the child or a family member if needed at a later time. On the other hand, Carol felt good about the fact that it could be potentially lifesaving for a patient with leukemia or any other type of blood cancer who needed a stem cell transplant and had no donor available. Searching the Internet, Carol learned that public cord blood banks needed more donations from certain ethnic groups, especially African Americans, Hispanics, and Asians. That caught her attention since she is Hispanic.

Since Carol didn't know what to do at this point, she decided to talk to her obstetrician about it and get her advice. She was surprised however when Dr. Bauer told her that she was not too familiar with the different options or the pros and cons of public and private cord blood banking. She just remembered that she had seen statements issued by professional organizations, the American Association of Pediatrics and the American Medical Association that discouraged private cord blood banking and was in favor of public banking. She promised Carol that she would speak with a colleague at the hospital where she worked, who was a specialist in bone marrow and stem cell transplant.

When Carol saw Dr. Bauer again, she was now thirty-two weeks pregnant and was anxious to learn more about the two cord-blood banking options. Dr. Bauer admitted that she was somewhat embarrassed that she did not know more about it, but mentioned that many of her colleagues don't seem to have a lot of detailed knowledge about the option of cord blood banking. Some admitted that they don't even mention it to the expectant mother.

PUBLIC CORD BLOOD BANKING

When the mother decides to have the cord blood donated to a public bank, she will have to get some extra blood tests done toward the end of the pregnancy to make sure she is free of any transmittable infections. The mother to be will also have to fill out a questionnaire similar to the one that is required prior to donating blood.

In order for a woman to donate cord blood to a public bank, the hospital must have a contractual relationship with a cord blood bank that is part of the National Marrow Donor Program (NMDP). This allows transplant physicians who search for a stem cell donor for a patient through the NMDP (Be the Match) database to look for a suitable cord blood unit. This can only be done if the cord blood has been stored with a bank that is affiliated with the NMDP.

Currently only about thirty public cord blood banks in the United States are part of this network, but the number is growing. About 100,000 cord blood units have been stored and are listed through the NMDP registry and the target number is around 150,000. A list of the about 200 NMDP-affiliated hospitals that accept cord blood donations can be found at www.parentsguidecordblood.org. This Web site also has some useful general information for prospective parents.

If the hospital is *not* affiliated with the NMDP, the mother to be can request a cord blood collection kit from the NMDP. The collection kit has about the size of a small microwave and contains a cord blood collection kit, and the necessary tubes and syringes for the doctor to collect the cord blood. After delivery, the cord blood from the baby is shipped to Cryobanks International www.cryo-intl.com/enroll/donating, a contract cord blood bank for the NMDP.

Not all collected cord blood collections will be stored in a public bank. If there are not enough stem cells in a collection (usually 900 million cells are the minimum), a public bank may not store the blood and instead release the cells for research or discard the unit. Unfortunately less than half of all collections submitted to public cord blood banks will get stored because they do not reach the target cell number. There are ways of maximizing the yield of a collection that are largely dependent on the experience of the obstetrician or the midwife. The birth weight of the baby, the time of cord clamping after delivery, and length of labor also have an impact on how many cells can be collected. Collecting cord blood involves extra paperwork and extra time in the delivery room. Since there is no fee for collecting cord blood, some obstetricians may not be too motivated to take this extra step.

Public cord blood banks currently provide stem cells only to support a transplant for FDA-approved indications, that is to replace diseased or malfunctioning bone marrow. They are not used for any disorders that could potentially be treated with cord blood cells in the future such as certain heart diseases, diabetes, or for replacement of cartilage or bone. Despite these concerns and after talking to her family, Carol decided to donate her child's cord blood cells to a public bank. Since Carol is Hispanic, the chance that cord blood from her baby could help a patient in need of a transplant were indeed quite promising.

Although public cord blood banks receive some federal funding, they usually have a hard time breaking even financially. Before the collected cord blood unit can be stored, the cord blood banks have to run a battery of tests that cannot be billed to the mother's insurance and hence have to be covered by the cord blood bank. The mother's blood and the cord blood have to be tested to exclude any infectious diseases or congenital blood abnormalities such as thalassemia or sickle cell disease. Also tissue typing (HLA typing) has to be performed on the blood cells.

This information is then entered into the central database of the NMDP. Together the testing of the mother's blood and the processing of the blood cost around

$1,500 per unit. This is one reason why public banks discard rather than freeze and store suboptimal collections. How do the cord blood banks make money or break even—by selling the cord blood unit to a transplant center for use with a patient. The average charge for a cord blood unit is about $35,000 and this amount is billed to the requesting hospital that in turn will invoice the patient's insurance.

Carol had questions about the technical details of cord blood donation—was there a risk for the baby or for the mother and was it painful or inconvenient? Dr. Bauer explained that "the collection of cord blood after delivery is without risk for the mother but requires a few extra steps by the obstetrician. After delivery of the baby, the umbilical cord is clamped as usual, and the baby is separated (cut) from it. Then the placenta is delivered as it is normally done and placed on a stand to allow the blood from the placenta to flow down into the cord. The vein of the cord is punctured at the bottom and the blood is drained into a sterile blood-collection bag.

The cord blood collection will not interfere with the care of the mother or the baby and does not pose any harm for either. The blood is then send to the contract cord blood storage facility, where it is processed. Upon arrival at the cord blood bank and before it can be frozen, the blood has to be checked to see if it contains enough stem cells and is free of any contamination. It is then stored in a special plastic bags (figure 6) in a liquid nitrogen tank at very cold tempartures (-320° F)

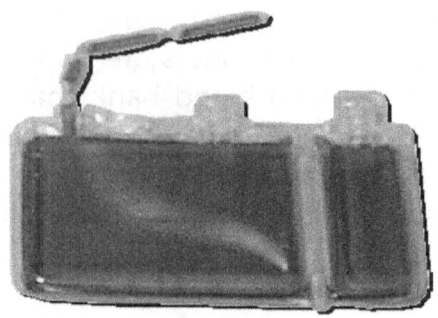

Figure 6

The cord blood is stored in a plastic bag. This particular one has a larger chamber that can keep about 75 percent of the volume and a smaller one with 25 percent of the collection. Both chambers are separated so that the stem cells can be used at different occasions and possibly for different indications, for example if expansion of the smaller volume if required for a second transplant. The bag also contains little attachments with small amounts of blood that can be cut off and the cord blood can be retested before it is given to the patient.

PRIVATE CORD BLOOD BANKING

Private or family cord blood banks have been around for much longer than public banks. Over 400,000 cord blood units are stored worldwide in private banks. They require an upfront processing fee (between $1,500 and $2,000) and an annual storage fee ($100 and 200). Recently some *hybrid* cord blood banks have sprung up that divide the cord blood collection and freeze it in two separate portions—one for public use if needed, and the other for use by the child or family member. However, unless scientists figure out how to expand and multiply the stem cells, the number in either chamber will be insufficient for transplant and even for regenerative medicine.

Most professional medical societies and most transplant physicians consider private banking a business model that capitalizes on the hopes of parents that these cells could be used at some point in the future in case the child develops a life-threatening blood cancer. The critics of family banking continue to be quite vocal. Unfortunately their critique also reflects some misconception and insufficient attention to the evolving research in stem cell biology. It doesn't take into consideration the spectrum of emerging indications for the use of cord blood stem cells that are mentioned in an earlier chapter. Most importantly, cord blood stem cells represent an excellent source of *early* stem cells that have long telomers and among other advantages, represent ideal cells to be used to generate induced pluripotent stem (iPS) cells (see chapter XIII) and at some point may be a good source of cloning tissues and perhaps organs for the original donor.

The critics are certainly correct that it is a remote possibility that the stored cord blood cells will ever be used in case the child develops leukemia or any other disease treatable by a bone marrow stem cell transplant.

Calculations predict that the likelihood of using a privately stored cord blood unit for transplant of a blood cancer is about 1:100,000. Even more relevant than these calculations is the question whether these cells are a suitable source of stem cells in case the child develops leukemia.

It clearly would be much better to use stem cells from a sibling or unrelated donor to have the benefit of the new donor immune system (the graft versus leukemia effect) transferred by the donor's bone marrow stem cells. Most importantly, the genetic predisposition to develop leukemia may already be anchored in the baby's genes before birth. Hence it would not make sense to use those stored cord blood cells. This seems to be the case especially for childhood leukemia that develops in the first years of life.

Dr. Bauer told Carol about some children, who at an early age, came down with acute leukemia. When their chromosomes were analyzed, they all had an abnormality involving an exchange between the chromosomes number four and number eleven. Fortuitously, these children had a drop of blood stored from the time of their birth for the Guthrie test. Some decades ago, the pediatrician Dr. Guthrie developed a simple blood test to detect a congenital metabolic disorder. Every newborn had to give a drop of blood after birth that was put on a piece of filter paper. These were kept over the decades and allowed researchers to go back and look for leukemia genes in those blood drops.

Since changes in the chromosomes four and eleven are common in leukemia, these findings confirmed that the children had their leukemia already predetermined in their genes. The use of their cord blood stem cells for transplant would have been detrimental and likely would have caused an immediate recurrence of their leukemia.

The opinions are somewhat split as to what happens when children develop leukemia later in life. It is possible that those "late" leukemias develop because of some environmental factors that we cannot exactly pinpoint at this time. Genetic abnormalities carried over from birth may not play a role in the manifestation of the disease. It is also less likely that other bone marrow and lymph cancers like myeloma and lymphoma that can develop later in life are anchored in our genes at the time of birth and are more likely the result of environmental factors.

Cord blood stem cells stored in a private bank, however, can be used for a sibling if needed. As we have calculated before, there is about a 25 percent chance that the sibling is matched with the cord blood donor. Parents and other relatives are generally not sufficiently tissue matched to receive the stored cord blood unit of their child as a transplant source in case a bone marrow or blood cancer strikes the family member.

Private cord blood banks can play an important role for direct donations. When a child has come down with leukemia and there is no brother or sister for bone marrow stem cell donation, if the parents are expecting another child, they can store the cord blood of the newborn. Again, there is a 25 percent chance that the new baby will be tissue matched with the sibling. Modern technology now allows testing for the HLA tissue type of the unborn child early during the pregnancy. Some parents may decide to carry out the pregnancy only if a baby in the womb has the desired tissue type. Such genetic selection is controversial from an ethical point as it can involve an abortion. Since chances are only 25 percent that the baby will have a compatible tissue type with the sick child, such an approach can theoretically lead to several abortions before the "right" child has been conceived. It becomes even more controversial when in vitro fertilization is involved to select for the "right" baby.

How long can cord blood stem cells be kept in the freezer and remain functional after thawing ? As far as research can tell us, they are probably good for a long time, maybe even forever. Although we may no longer use today's technology to do a stem cell transplant for leukemia and other blood cancers, we likely will continue to use cord blood as a source of early stem cells for example for regenerative medicine. Scientists likely will be able to isolate the stem cells and grow them in larger numbers, manipulate them, and possibly even change their genetic makeup.

Although the expansion of stem cells from cord blood will become possible in the next five to ten years, it is still important to maximize the number of cord blood stem cells that are collected at birth. Collections may have sufficient numbers to support a transplant for a small child, but there are frequently not enough stem cells in a cord blood unit for an adolescent or adult patient. In contrast to public cord blood banks that will not store these suboptimal collections, private cord blood banks have a lower cutoff, allowing more donated units to be stored. The argument for keeping those collections is that technologies to expand the stem cell pool will become available at some point in the future.

Recently, researchers in Seattle have succeeded in tricking stem cells into making more of their own by adding a factor that activates certain genes in stem cells and essentially turns on their engine to divide and multiply. A similar effect can be accomplished with "reprogramming" cord blood stem cells to become induced pluripotent stem cells (iPS, see chapter XIII), which resemble embryonic stem cells and can be driven to develop certain tissues. However playing with the genetic makeup of a cell can be problematic, and the FDA has placed strict regulatory requirements on it. This technology is at least five to ten years away before it can be tested in humans provided it continues to show promise in animal models.

A more readily available technology of promoting the take of limited number of cord blood stem cells is by adding helper cells that provide a nurturing environment for the cord blood stem cells. First observations in patients suggest that the mesenchymal stem cells (MSC) could be such a cell when transplanted together with the cord blood stem cells. Since MSC can be obtained relatively easily either from bone marrow of any healthy person or from the umbilical cord itself (the jelly cells) at the time of delivery, the combined storage of cord blood and jelly cells as a MSC source is getting some traction and more and more private cord blood banks are offering this service in addition to cord blood banking.

Carol wanted to know how many transplants had actually been performed with cord blood cells from private banks. Dr. Bauer explained that an exact number is difficult to calculate as these numbers are not readily published, but that the number was somewhere around 300.

Most private cord blood banks still advertise that the foremost reason why parents should store their baby's cord blood is for a transplant in case the child develops a bone marrow or blood cancer. However as we calculated earlier, this fairly remote possibility should not be the central argument that private cord blood banks make in favor of storage. Cord blood contains several highly potent stem cells that can give rise to several tissues in the body. There is already plenty of evidence from animal studies that cells from cord blood have unique healing and regenerative properties (chapter IX). Not only contain cord blood cells the precious hematopoietic stem cells (HSC) that can produce new blood cells but they also contain additional stem cells types like mesenchymal and entdothelial *stem* cells that can contribute to the beneficial effects described in chapter IX.

In addition, cord blood cells have long telomers (chapter IX) and are young cells. They are ideally suited to manipulation and engineering at some point in the future when those technologies become available. Turning them into induced pluripotent stem cells (iPS cells) with embryonic stem cell like features is just one option. There is also the evolving field of regenerative medicine that seems to favor cord blood cells as they are the patient's own stem cells and represent young cells with a genetic makeup that has not been exposed to environmental factors that potentially can alter and affect genes.

Private cord blood banks are denounced by most, if not all, professional medical organizations. Most of these opinions are based on a lack of understanding of what cord blood stem cells and stem cells from other tissue sources could provide to an individual, especially in the field of regenerative medicine, in the near future.

A fairly typical recommendation recently issued by the European Group on Ethics shows the problem and at times confusing wording, these organizations struggle with: *"the legitimacy of commercial cord blood banks for autologous use should be questioned as they sell a service, which has presently no real use regarding therapeutic options. Thus they promise more than they can deliver. The activities of such banks raise serious ethical questions."* This wording is confusing to future parents and in fact not very helpful especially when the society's statement goes on to say: *"if in the future regenerative medicine developed in such a way that using autologous stem cells became possible, then the fact to have one's own cord blood being stored at birth could increase the chance of having access to new therapies."* Unfortunately for many people it may be too late because their early stem cells may not have been banked.

Another argument that is frequently mentioned is that numerous patients with leukemia or blood cancer are in need of a stem cell donor but can't find a suitable donor in the public cord blood registry. Hence it is irresponsible to bank cord blood for private or family use and the mother should instead donate to a public cord blood bank. The reality though is that sufficient cord blood units from Caucasians are stored in public banks and that the real need is to get African Americans, Asians, and Native Indians to enroll and save the cord blood stem cells.

However, some banking companies are pushing the business aspect too much. At times promises are made that cannot be backed by available data. This leaves the industry open to criticism that only further confuses the consumer.

On the other hand it is not helpful to patients and consumers either when adult stem cell storage is categorically discredited.

Cord blood is just one source of adult stem cells that have been banked for more than twenty years. As additional stem cells sources are discovered, the service of storing these cells for a fee will be offered by a rapidly rising number of companies. As we have seen in the previous chapter, baby and adult teeth, menstrual blood, umbilical cord, placenta, amniotic fluid, and peripheral blood are already stored for potential future use.

STEM CELLS FOR RESCUE AFTER RADIATION EXPOSURE

Since our society is increasingly concerned about mass radiation as acts of bio-terrorism, would stem cell transplants potentially save lives? Bone marrow certainly is the tissue in our body that is most sensitive to radiation and blood counts may drop to levels where the risk of bleeding (low platelets) or infections (low white cells) is high. We know, however, from the nuclear accident in Chernobyl in 1984, how difficult it is to do bone marrow stem cell transplants under those circumstances particularly when only unrelated not well matched donors are available.

None of the victims of in the Chernobyl accident who were given an unrelated bone marrow stem cell transplant survived. For once the transplanted bone marrow stem cells were not well tissue matched. The National Marrow Donor Program (NMDP) was still in its infancy and did not have a pool of well-tissue-typed volunteer donors. Cord blood stem cells that require less perfect matching with the recipient and could have resulted in better outcome but were not available at that time. Rejection of the transplanted cells and GvHD were major problems in transplanted recipients.

Another concern in radiation accidents is the damage to other organs that can affect their function. If those patients undergo a bone marrow stem cell transplant, they will need a host of drugs to prevent rejection and GvHD, and to prevent and treat infections. Those interventions require stable organ function. From that perspective, having the patient's own stem cells stored would remove some of those problems as rejection or GvHD would not occur.

The government has asked the stem cell company Osiris to stockpile their mesenchymal stem cells (MSC) to be available in case of radiation exposure. This was done with the intent that the MSC can be given to victims to help healing organs that may be damaged from radiation. With our expanding knowledge about induced pluripotent stem cells (iPS), these cells may also be used as a platform to generate new blood cells.

XII.
STEM CELLS FOR YOUR PET?

A whole new industry has sprung up. Since veterinary medicine is less regulated and novel treatments can be given to animals without heavy involvement of the Federal Drug Agency (FDA), animals have received stem cells treatments, mostly in form of mesenchymal stem cells (MSC). For example, if racehorses experience some form of tendon, ligament, or joint injury, it could potentially mean a loss of significant prize money. Mesenchymal stem cells (MSC) can be obtained from fat tissue. About two tablespoons of fat are aspirated from the back of the injured horse and sent in a container to a special laboratory that will grow the MSC cells and send them back to the horse's veterinarian for injection at the injured site. Another company uses MSC from bone marrow obtained from the horse's chest bone. More than 1,500 race horses have been treated using this process and follow-up data suggests that, compared with conventional treatment, the incidence of re-injury over the years is reduced by at least 50 percent. Traditional therapies transplanting tendons obtained from dead horses are both less efficient and have a high risk of re-injury.

Some dogs, like German shepherds, are known to develop arthritis in their knees relatively early in their lives, which can be painful and restricts their mobility. Biotech companies are offering the same treatment that has worked for racehorses now for the treatment of arthritis in dogs. The veterinarian obtains some fat tissue (usually from the abdomen) or bone marrow from the dog, and sends it to the laboratory where MSC are generated. The cells are then returned to the veterinarian for injection into the joint.

Since the MSC are the cells that are responsible for the healing, other more accessible MSC sources will be used in the future. Mesenchymal stem cells (MSC) from the umbilical cord or placenta contain millions of those cells. Since MSC can be given to other animals without fear of rejection, MSC for regenerative treatments can come from a bank that have stored these MSC rich tissues.

XIII.
EMBRYONIC STEM CELLS: HYPE OR REAL OPPORTUNITY?

The California-based biotech company Geron is one of the driving forces to bring embryonic stem cells into the clinical practice. Their studies in rats have shown that treated animals regained their ability to walk and run after spinal cord injury, although they continued to limp. To prepare those stem cells, Geron scientists force embryonic stem cells to develop in the direction of nerve precursor cells that are then injected around the lesion in the spinal cord. A small clinical trial (planned are 10 patients) just opened and will mostly look at the safety of injecting stem cells into the spinal cord. Only patients with a recent spinal injury will be eligible.

What are embryonic stem cells ? After the egg has combined with a sperm cell, it begins to divide. In the early stages an *inner cell mass* (about five days after fertilization) is formed. This inner cell mass, called *blastocyts* is then removed using fine instruments and placed into a culture dish where they can be maintained and produce more of their own. The end product is a stem cell line that consists of identical cells. By adding certain proteins and hormones, the embryonic stem cells can be coaxed into different body cells and produce tissue specific cells.

Embryonic stem cells are considered *pluripotent* because they have the ability to transform into *any* body cell type, since they have the full genetic program to do so. This is different for adult stem cells that can only produce one type of body cell (unipotent) or at most different types of specialized cells (multipotent) but never an entire organ that is composed of different cells with varying functions.

The National Institutes of Health (NIH) has been very cognizant of the opinions and emotions that surround embryonic stem cell research. In order to get embryonic stem cells, an early stage embryo consisting of a ball of cells is sacrificed. These fertilized embryos are usually obtained from reproductive centers that have many unused embryos from parents in the freezer. Those parents gave consent to give up the fertilized eggs and make them available for research. The NIH has drafted strict guidelines for the generation of these lines and an administrative review at the NIH closely examines the submitted lines to make sure they adhere to the NIH guidelines in terms of the informed consent process.

During the Bush administration, research with embryonic stem cells was restricted and no government grants and monies were available. Scientists could only work with embryonic stem cells when they had private funding available and this restricted research mostly to biotech-nolgy and pharmaceutical companies. Although this has changed under the current administration, this topic is so contentious that it can be expected that decisions on federal funding may go back and forth.

Why are embryonic stem cells touted as so promising? It is believed that they potentially can grow into any type of tissue and even an entire organ. However, that is likely more than decades away as methods have to be developed to accomplish the three dimensional structure of an organ along with generating all the different specialized cells that make up an organ. Scientists will have to learn to turn the right genes on and off at the right time to create a functional organ.

The body has over 200 different cell types, and scientists will first have to understand the factors and pathways that govern the differentiation of embryonic stem cells into a specific cell type. This remains poorly understood. Even if large numbers of specific cells can be generated, they have to be properly assembled and, for example, in the case of a blood vessel, they have to have the mechanical strength to resist the impact of the blood flow. Since they are generated from a genetically different individual, rejection of the transplanted tissue can also be problem. Finally, the problem of tumor formation that can originate from those cells need to be resolved. After all embryonic stem cells are universal cells, and the researcher's manipulations have just "tamed" them. There is always the possibility that they can break free and among other things cause cancerous growth.

The path to developing embryonic stem cells can have unanticipated roadblocks. Scientists were able to generate sperm from embryonic stem cells in mice that could even fertilize an egg. That seems like good news for infertile couples, but unfortunately, the offspring created with those sperm cells had some unexpected and serious organ abnormities and deformities. This just shows that it can be challenging to control and direct the large genetic program of embryonic stem cells.

Assuming that it is ten to fifteen years later, and scientists have learned to prevent tumor formation and rejection, than one near term goal for embryonic stem cell research could be to generate insulin-producing islet cells that can be implanted into the body to treat diabetes. Those cells don't require a complicated tissue structure. The government has made funding available to explore the potential of embryonic stem cells to differentiate into those islet cells.

THE FLUENT BORDERS TO CLONING

In 1938 the German pathologist Hans Spemann made an exciting observation that should be remembered as the first proof of reprogramming human cells. He removed the genetic material from the fertilized egg of a salamander and then replaced it with the DNA (the genes) obtained from the body cells of another but much older animal. Despite the different genes and the fact that the genes came from an older cell, the egg could still develop into an entire salamander. The genes of the older cell still had the entire genetic information available and were able to unblock that information, reverting back to an embryonic like cell that were able to program a "new" animal.

Cloning is another way of creating identical cells from a single cell (figure 7). The genetic material, the DNA of a normal human female egg is removed and instead the DNA obtained from a body cells of the individual to be cloned is inserted into that egg; this essentially replaces the genetic "program" of the egg with the other person's genes. This is also known as *nuclear transfer*. When these cells divide, they form an embryo and like with embryonic stem cells, the inner cell mass (*blastocyst*) can be removed and grown in the plastic dish to produce patient specific tissues. This is *therapeutic cloning*.

Much hope is placed on therapeutic cloning. Drug companies believe that this technology would allow testing new drug candidates before they are given to patients, better defining their efficacy profile and also possible side effects. In that case, the DNA from a patient with a specific disease would be transferred to an egg to generate patient-specific tissue through nuclear transfer. Pharmaceutical companies are embracing this technology as it would make it possible to screen large numbers of candidate compounds and identify the ones that are worth further development.

Scientists, however, are still somewhat skeptical, how well cells made in a test tube really resemble their adult counterparts. They tend to resemble more fetal cells rather than adult forms of brain, blood, or heart cells. How well can a reprogrammed cell from a person reflect what a heart cell may have experienced throughout a lifetime, especially in late onset diseases with multiple contributing factors, such as heart disease? How well can a cell in a plastic dish really simulate the effects of an unlucky inheritance possibly combined with decades of bad eating and poor physical activity?

Instead of removing the inner cell mass from the blastocyte for therapeutic cloning, the egg can be implanted back into the uterus (womb). It can develop into a full embryo and ultimately into an individual that is essentially a carbon copy of the person who donated the DNA. This is *reproductive cloning*, a highly controversial research. We all know Dolly, the sheep that was created in 1997 by reproductive cloning. Since Dolly, several other animals have been cloned. Although the process sounds quite straightforward, the resulting animals can have a number of health problems, one of them is premature aging which occurs because the telomers that sit on the ends of chromosomes and that guard the aging of the cells, were already much shorter in the mature body cell.

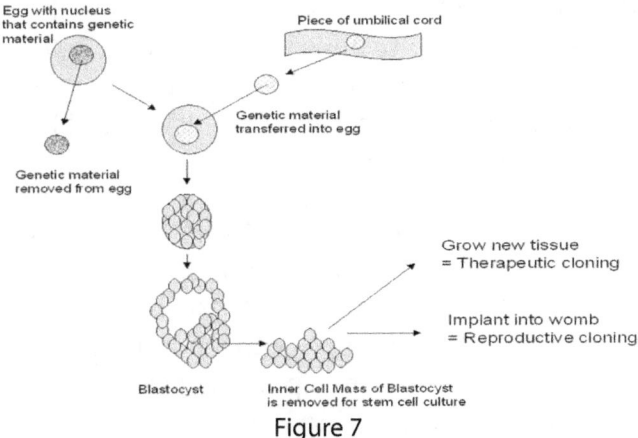

Figure 7

Principle of **nuclear transfer** and **cloning**: the genetic material located in the nucleus of a cell is removed from a female egg and replaced by the nucleus with the genetic material of another cell (in this case a from the umbilical cord). After a few cell divisions, the *blastocyst* is formed whose *inner cell mass* can be grown out into a donor-specific stem cell line (therapeutic cloning). If the blastocyst is implanted into the womb, it grows into a new individual—identical (a clone) to the donor (reproductive cloning).

MAKING EMBRYONIC LIKE STEM CELLS WITHOUT EMBRYOS

It will remain speculation as to how much the initial ban on federally funded work with embryonic stem cells during the Bush administration possibly stimulated the creativity of scientists to develop alternative models. Several years ago, researchers found a way of making embryonic-like stem cells. Interestingly, there are some similarities to the observations that Spemann made in salamanders almost 100 years ago. Fully differentiated "older" cells can turn into embryonic-like stem cells that now have the entire genetic equipment to behave like embryonic cells. Scientists can take any body cell and activate certain genes that are crucial to embryonic stem cells. This cell will be reprogrammed and become iPS.

Here is how it works: a human cell (even a skin cell will suffice) is treated with certain chemicals that will activate key genes that lay dormant in the cell. By activating the right genes, the cell reverts back to a primitive embryonic stage and now can be manipulated like an embryonic stem cell. The reprogramming is accomplished by forcing adult body cells to produce proteins that are key to the pluripotent behavior of embryonic stem cells.

Initially scientists were using viruses to shuttle genes into the cells that would do the reprogramming of the host cell. These genes are typical for young stem cells and have funny names like Oct, Sox, KL4, and Myc. The transfer of viruses into a cell is not without risk because where the genes will insert into the normal genome cannot be controlled. If they insert at the wrong place in the genome, they can activate cancer genes that every person has in their genes and which usually remain silent. More recently scientists have discovered that some chemicals and molecules seem to accomplish the same effect as the viruses, and this is a much safer method.

What scientists have learned from iPS cells and what Spemann already had concluded from his salamander experiments was that every body cell carries the full genetic information. The difference to an embryonic stem cell is that certain of its genes are suppressed and deactivated to allow the adult stem cell to function only in a particular direction and to produce daughter cells. However, those deactivated genes can be restored and then a normal human body cell can behave like an embryonic stem cell.

iPS cells actually look and act quite similar to embryonic stem cells. Since iPS cells are not derived from embryos, they don't carry the baggage of ethical concerns surrounding the use of embryonic stem cells. All of this then makes one question whether we really need embryonic stem cells. Despite the startling discoveries with iPS cells, recent research is showing that they are not quite of the same quality as embryonic stem cells and that the iPS cells tend to age and die earlier. This should not come as a surprise as body cells have shorter telomers than embryonic or fetal cells. The lifespan of the newly created iPS cells may be limited by the age of the original cell.

Biotechnology companies hope to use both embryonic and iPS cells to screen new drug candidates, study organ development, and possibly grow tissues for transplantation that would not be rejected. However formidable challenges remain even with iPS cells. Like regular embryonic stem cells, iPS cells can form tumors when implanted in tissue. The rejection is less of an issue as these cells would be autologous cells, coming from the same person. Using skin cells or any other body cells from a patient carries the additional risk that a biologically "old" cell is propagated. These cells contain more DNA abnormalities caused by exposure to sunlight, toxins, and the likelihood of errors in making more DNA copies during the cause of a lifetime.

In addition scientists have found that even after reprogramming, iPS cells retain the "footprint" of the tissue from which they were derived. In order to overcome the problem of age (shorter telomers) scientists are now using cells from fetal tissue, the placenta or from umbilical cord blood.

XIV.

STEM CELLS: THE BUSINESS

Since the term *stem cell* is somewhat reminiscent of creation – there is the hope that stem cells can already or soon will be able to cure many of the ailments humans encounter in their lifetime. Numerous stem cell biotechnology companies have sprung up. Some will survive because they are doing reputable research and testing their stem cell product in well-designed clinical trials. At the end of this chapter is a summary of stem cell trials that are currently enrolling patients in North America.

However, there is the large unregulated grey area of stem cell medicine that happens predominantly in countries outside of the United States. Dubious clinics offer stem cell infusions often with unproven benefit and pray on the hope of vulnerable patients. These clinics and their treatments are not regulated by the FDA, and there is no FDA assurance that the treatments are safe. Although the public at times may view the FDA as impeding the rapid access to new treatments, this process is important to prevent harm to the public and the individual.

The history of the FDA goes back to 1906, when Congress passed the Food and Drug Act, which made it illegal to distribute misbranded or adulterated foods, drinks, and drugs across state lines. In 1937 Sulfanilamide was hailed as the first drug for strep throat and gonorrhea formulated into an elixir. The liquid formulation however contained antifreeze, and it killed 107 people, mostly children. This happened because an earlier law did not require the drug's manufacturer to test the formulation for *safety* before it was sold. For this and many other reasons, the FDA is now an important safety check for new drugs and treatments.

The FDA has set a high bar for stem cell treatments. Applications for using stem cells in humans "have to have compelling data in order to move them into human trials." Clearly the FDA's wariness is due to uncertainty about the effect of stem cells on the body especially when it comes to their potential of causing cancer. In the United States, some stem cell companies are nearing human trials with embryonic stem cells; this is largely uncharted territory for stem cell therapies. In addition to demonstrating safety of their stem cell product, the companies also have to assure that treated patients are monitored for the rest of their lives.

Stem cell clinics abroad offer treatments that in most cases have not been validated as being safe and effective. The source for those adult stem cells can vary and may include bone marrow, cord blood, or fetal cells. A whole spectrum of diseases is treated with stem cell infusions ranging from autism and cerebral palsy to spinal cord injury and diabetes. The site of injection of stem cells can vary; for example, for the treatment of Parkinson, these cells are injected either into the brain fluid through a lumbar puncture or directly implanted into the brain during a stereotactic operation. Although I some cases the patient's own stored cord blood cells are injected, frequently the cells come from an unrelated donor.

Patients from all over the world come to those clinics for treatments, some of which are outright fraudulent and not based on any scientific data. Despite the fact that thousands of patients have been "treated," no publications in recognized journals are available that would allow the medical community to get a better understanding of those unproven treatments. The clinics and institutions usually list some anecdotal patient stories on their Web sites. Apart from the fact that only stories of those patients who may have had some improvement will be listed, it is well known that some disorders can spontaneously improve. It is also quite well known that any medical procedure can have a placebo effect that gives the patient the impression of improvement and "success."

Stem cell treatments abroad can be expensive and are generally not paid for by U.S. insurance. With an average of $20,000 per treatment, this can be a significant source of income not only for the clinic itself but also for the country where the clinic operates. The Chinese health care company Beike claims that is has treated over 6,000 patients. The company runs more than twenty clinics in China and Thailand and claims to have received funding from the Chinese government, essentially using this financial support as a seal of approval for their unapproved treatments.

Under international pressure, the Chinese Health Ministry announced that it would take steps to regulate medical stem cell technologies and treatments. Hospitals around the country were supposed to either stop providing unproven treatments or apply to the ministry for approval. Although this sounds like a step in the right direction, serious questions remain as to how and whether those regulations will be enforced. The fines for breaching the regulation are about $1,000, and it is unlikely that this relatively small fee will deter large operations from offering those therapies.

Some of the experimental treatments can be outright dangerous. Recently a tumor was found in the brain of a boy who had stem cells injected into his brain to cure a brain disorder. The treatment was performed in a clinic in Russia. It appears that the injected stem cells came from the brain of an aborted fetus, and studies confirmed that the tumor originated from the injected cells (www.isscr. org/public/briefings/danger.html).

Recently the International Society for Stem Cell Research (ISSCR) issued "Guidelines for the Transplantation of Stem Cell Research," which can be found on their Web site (www.isscr.org/clinical_trans/index.cfm). This is an important and highly needed initiative as the number of stem cell clinics offering treatments in countries where the regulations are lax and lenient has boomed. The ISSCR will even go one step further and requires some proof that the treatments are based on previously completed animal studies or assurance that the study is conducted on an approved protocol from institutions offering these therapies. If that is not the case, these clinics and institutions will be blacklisted.

In the case of China, there are some attempts for the country to gain more recognition as a player especially in the field of regenerative medicine. A number of properly conducted clinical trials are underway for conditions like heart disease, restricted blood flow to the limbs, and spinal cord injuries.

One may wonder why patients must go to other countries for treatments that are considered experimental. One of the reasons is that our litigious environment has gradually discouraged physicians from initiating more complex and risky clinical trials. A young physician at the beginning of his or her career will not venture into a field that is controversial and for which it would be difficult to get funding. Established investigators on the other hand are concerned their reputation may suffer or they might lose grant funding.

Some stem cell products can enter the U.S. market if they are labeled as nutrients, cosmetics, or vitamins rather than drugs. The FDA does not monitor items in those categories as closely. An example is a facial cream made from cord blood stem cells advertised to rejuvenate the skin. The cream's active ingredients include "Human Stem Cell Conditioned Media." The company has a proprietary method to isolate and culture mesenchymal stem cells (MSC) from frozen umbilical cord cells. In culture these MSC produce a number of proteins that are secreted into the culture medium that is then further processed and added to a cream base as the primary ingredient. It is hard to measure any benefit of this and similar products. Controlled studies to show efficacy are not required to sell those topical products.

Another example of marketing an unproven stem cell treatment is advertised as a pill that will increase the bone marrow stem cells in blood. According to the company, these cells help to rejuvenate and heal the body tissue that undergoes wear and tear daily. This ultimately will lead to well-being and better health.

Assuming the medication does indeed increase the number of circulating blood stem cells, it is unclear why such an increase would be of any benefit. The bone marrow already sends out millions of cells into the blood every day, so would such a small increase for a short period of time really make a difference?

Moreover, healthy volunteers who donate bone marrow or blood stem cells for a patient in need will receive a drug (Neupogen) that significantly increases the number of bone marrow stem cells in the blood. This stem cell mobilization allows sufficient stem cells to be obtained from the blood for transplantation when the bone marrow is affected by leukemia. None of those donors ever reported that they were feeling any better afterward.

XV.

STEM CELL TRIALS IN NORTH AMERICA

A number of stem cell trials are open for enrollment in the United States and Canada. The number of clinical trials in countries around the world is just skyrocketing as most countries have less stringent regulations for conducting clinical trials than the United States.

The early studies in humans are phase I trials. The purpose of those is to determine if the new treatment is safe and if there are any unexpected side effects. A *phase I* trial may start at a low dose or cell number. Usually three or four patients are enrolled at each dose level, and if no side effects are observed within a certain time period, the next cohort of patients will receive a higher dose. Such a dose-escalation study usually enrolls nine to fifteen patients before it is closed. Although some beneficial effect may occur for an individual enrolled on a phase one trial, this cannot be guaranteed and is not the primary goal of the trial.

Phase II studies will look at whether the treatment has some benefit for the patient. The dose of the drug or the number of cells used for the study will be based on what was determined to be safe in a phase one trial. Although those studies are important, their outcome will not tell whether there is any improvement over current standard therapy, which is the objective of *a phase III* trial. These trials are usually done in a randomized fashion, which means that the assignment to an experimental or standard treatment (or no treatment) is by chance and is determined by a computer. If it is a blind study, neither patients nor their physicians know whether they received the active drug.

Once the clinical trials are completed, the company producing the drug can apply for a "label." The FDA will review the file with the safety and efficacy data and can then approve the treatment for a specific indication. The approval requires that the new treatment shows some benefit for patients in the phase III comparison. However there may be some diseases in which it is difficult to conduct a large phase three trial and for which only limited treatment options are available. In those situations, the company can apply for orphan drug status, which gives financial and regulatory incentives to companies to develop these treatments. Orphan status speeds up the approval process.

Research in regenerative medicine is very active, and we read every day about remarkable progress that scientists make. However the path from curing a disease in a laboratory animal and being able to take that observation into a clinical trial can take years and requires substantial financial commitment. Stem cell trials are much more expensive than trials testing a pill, and there are still tremendous challenges in developing a stem cell therapy into a clinical grade product. Manufacturing a pill or suspension requires a chemical plant, as well as packaging and distribution along established infrastructures. In contrast, getting a stem cell product from the manufacturer to the patient requires different scale-up technologies, facilities, and distribution mechanisms that essentially need to get established for each different stem cell product. Among other things, this will make stem cell therapies much more expensive.

Furthermore, a pill or suspension can be tested in a batch at the plant of the pharmaceutical company for purity and sterility before it is sent out to pharmacies. In contrast, any cell therapy product has to undergo individual release testing before it is given to the patient. This requires that viability and sterility testing is sent to the laboratory of the dispensing hospital and only if those results come back negative, can the product be given. Because of the limited lifespan of stem cells, they have to be shipped immediately unless they can be frozen and shipped in a frozen state. In many cases the personnel at the hospital also need to get special training as to how to prepare the stem cell product for infusion.

The following is a summary of ongoing clinical stem cell trials in North America offered for various diseases. Bone marrow stem cell transplant trials for treatment of bone marrow or blood cancers are not listed because most of them are considered standard of care and are offered at almost all academic medical centers.

Some major medical centers are able to conduct their own trials with stem cells that require access to a special laboratory facility that is frequently attached to the blood bank of the institution, where cell preparations can be performed according to FDA regulations. These facilities allow medical centers to prepare stem cells. However, since most stem cell trials are considered experimental at this point, the investigator will have to design a clinical protocol and have it approved by the institutional review board (IRB) that will look at feasibility of the treatment and more importantly whether it safeguards the patient. The protocol also contains a detailed informed consent that is written in lay language for the patient to sign before any treatment can be given. In addition to the scientific merit, the IRB will check if the treatment violates any ethics. Membership of this board is made up of a range of people with different backgrounds, including scientific peers, laypersons, and clergy.

For most stem cell trials, IRB approval will not suffice, and the investigator will have to file an investigational new drug (IND) application with the FDA, which will make sure that its standards are followed with regard to preparation and dispensing of the stem cell product. It will also assure that sufficient laboratory and animal data are available to justify the use of this particular stem cell preparation in humans. The FDA sets a high bar for stem cell treatments and expects that any stem cell based therapy would have to have very compelling data especially in animals in order to move into human trials. The FDA's wariness is due to uncertainty about stem cells effects on the body. While the treatments show promise, researchers do not yet have all the answers regarding the long-term effects of such treatments. In particular, tumors in the recipients continue to be a concern.

Biotechnology companies sponsor most of the stem cell treatment trials. These companies may have developed proprietary technologies to prepare stem cells. For example, they may use a special method to treat bone marrow stem cells, so that they become more specialized cells like nerve cells. In those cases, the company will identify institutions that will be able to conduct the trial and will also provide a clinical protocol. The company is also responsible for the paperwork with the FDA and for the monitoring of the study at the institution. The responsibility of the trial site is to properly conduct the study and collect all the data, which are considered the property of the company. In return, the company will pay a fee to the institution to cover the expenses for the trial and the rights to use the data.

The best way for a patient to identify a clinical trial is to log on to the NIH Web site (www.clinicaltrials.gov), which lists all current clinical trials. The listing on the government Web site does not necessarily mean that these trials are supported or approved by the NIH. Many of the stem cell studies are currently conducted abroad because of the different and often more lenient regulatory environment in some of the countries. Although this may be attractive to some patients seeking treatment, a thorough regulatory pathway also assures a higher degree of safety. Another web site with listing of trials is www.centerwatch.org.

There are a fair number of stem cells companies working on new stem cell treatments. Individuals reviewing these Web sites should be mindful that some of those sites might read as if the treatment is already available in clinical trials. Frequently they are only in the developmental stage, and it will take years for them to enter the clinic. Many of those company statements are "forward looking" and the text is more or less geared to attract investors. Text at the end usually serves as a disclaimer.

The following is a list of currently active stem cell trials by disease site. Since this is a rapidly advancing medical field, and although every effort was made to capture ongoing trials, the listing may not be complete. This summary however covers most of the diseases that represent active areas of clinical stem cell research.

PERIPHERAL ARTERY DISEASE

An impaired blood flow to the leg and foot (limb ischemia) is usually caused by a blockage of the arteries. Patients with this condition may experience intermittent or persistent severe pain in their lower extremities and may also develop severe tissue damage in the affected leg or foot. There are no drugs currently approved by the FDA for the treatment of this condition. For advanced critical limb ischemia, amputation of the affected limb is often the only available therapy option. Patients with diabetes are at higher risk for developing this disease at an early stage.

Several medical centers in the United States are part of a study called Harvest, which involves having bone marrow cells from the patient separated at the bedside and then injected into the muscle of the affected limb. This and other similar trials reported improved blood circulation and healing of ulcers even in diabetic patients.

The Center for Therapeutic Angiogenesis in Birmingham, Alabama, and Duke University Medical Center are injecting mesenchymal stem cells (MSC) into the affected leg. The stem cells come from the placenta and have been grown in a special bioreactor in large quantities (www.pluristem. com).

Northwestern University in Chicago (www.northwestern. edu) also offers a clinical trial where tissue-matched cord blood cells are injected into the muscle adjacent to the area of ischemia.

DIABETES

There are two types of diabetes: The most common form is type II, which manifests itself if the insulin producing islet cells in the pancreas are "exhausted" and no longer produce enough insulin to regulate the sugar level in blood. No stem cell treatment is available at this point although some biotech companies are attempting to generate new islet cells from bone marrow, cord blood stem cells, or even embryonic stem cells.

Type I diabetes affects mostly young adults and is also known as juvenile diabetes. This form of diabetes is caused by a self-destruction of the islet cells. Patients become dependent on insulin injections for the rest of their lives. In addition to the inconvenience of daily injection, diabetes patients also develop vascular complications relatively early in their lives, which is responsible for heart disease, stroke, blindness, nerve damage, and kidney impairment.

A few centers around the world are testing in clinical trials the infusion of autologous bone marrow stem cells after a round of chemotherapy and immune suppression of the patient. Scientists at Northwestern University have shown that this can lead to insulin independence in some patients while others may require less insulin. The problem with this trial is that it involves giving chemotherapy to an individual who does not suffer from a malignant disease. It is known that these drugs can affect healthy stem cells and may increase the chance of getting leukemia later in life.

Osiris (www.osiris.com) is sponsoring a multicenter trial across the United States in patients with newly diagnosed juvenile diabetes. Mesenchymal stem cells (MSC) obtained from healthy donors are infused if a patient has developed diabetes within a six-week window. The MSC are obtained from the bone marrow of healthy unrelated donors, and the recipient does not need immune suppression as MSC are not recognized by the immune system. This study is open at some twenty centers in the United States.

HEART ATTACK AND HEART FAILURE

A number of centers around the country are using the patients' own bone marrow cells for this stem cell treatment for the heart. About a cup of bone marrow is obtained from the patient's hipbone within the first days of the heart attack. The marrow is filtered to remove the red cells, and the remaining cells (containing stem cells) are either infused directly into the coronary arteries or injected into the affected heart tissue. These studies are designed to test whether this treatment can prevent or reduce symptoms related to heart damage that continue to develop following heart attack, including low pumping capacity, inflammation, and increased scar tissue.

Instead of injecting bone marrow cells, a preparation of mesenchymal stem cells (MSC) prepared form the bone marrow of healthy volunteer donors is also under study. Patients receive MSC (one time) within seven days of their attack. They are injected into the vein. Another approach of getting bone marrow cells to the affected area in the heart area is by injecting them into the artery that provides the area with blood. This is a more invasive approach, and it is currently not clear which form of stem cell administration is most beneficial.

Heart failure is a consequence of diminished blood flow to the heart that can occur after a heart attack or more chronically over time if the blood flow to a specific area of the heart is impeded. The heart muscle is damaged to the extent that it becomes dilated and has limited pump function. Patients on this trial receive MSC cells injected directly into the heart muscle.

SPINAL CORD INJURY

Some studies in mice and rats suggest some benefit from placing embryonic stem cells around the area of tissue injury. Scientists at the biotechnology company Geron have succeeded in creating some early nerve cells from embryonic stem cells. Ten patients will be treated in a phase I trial. The cells are placed in the area of the spinal cord injury. Only patients with a recent (< 14 days) spinal cord injury that occurred in the chest area, will be eligible.

PARKINSON DISEASE

Parkinson's disease is a relatively common disorder of brain cells that affects more than 2 percent of the population over sixty-five years of age. It is caused by a progressive degeneration and loss of brain cells that produce, the hormone dopamine, among other transmitters. Patients with Parkinson disease can develop uncontrollable shaking (tremor), stiffness (rigidity), and decreased mobility. Although it is hoped that Parkinson disease may be the first disease to be amenable to treatment using stem cell transplantation, so far no clinical trials in North America are underway.

LOU GEHRIG'S DISEASE

This is also known by its medical term as amyotrophic lateral sclerosis (ALS). This is progressive damage to nerve cells that occurs over time for unknown reasons. Patients become progressively paralyzed and die because their muscles cannot support breathing or any other life-supporting activity. ALS affects about 30,000 people in the United States with about 7,000 new diagnoses every year. Based on encouraging results in rats, the stem cells for this trial in humans are injected in the lower part of the spinal cord. This is a phase I trial to make sure that the injection of stem cells will not cause any damage. Twelve to eighteen patients will be enrolled. The trial is conducted at Emory University and the nerve stem cells are manufactured and provided by Neuralstem. The company obtains nerve stem cells from aborted fetuses and prepares them for injection. If the treatment is safe and works, the company plans to test these cells in other diseases involving nerve decay such as Huntington disease and spinal cord injury. The first few patients selected for this procedure will be those who are no longer able to walk.

STROKE

A stroke occurs when the blood flow leading to the brain is blocked or blood vessels in the brain rupture. No stem cell trial for stroke is open in the United States, but several medical centers around the world are offering the infusion of mesenchymal cells or bone marrow derived stem cells.

The British Biotech ReNeuron is about to begin a phase one trial in the United Kingdom for disabled stroke patients. Nerve stem cells are directly injected into the infarcted area of the brain. The nerve stem cells are obtained from a cell line that has been established from brain stem cells of an aborted fetus in 2003. The company tried to get permission from the FDA to conduct the trial in the United States, but the agency had problems with putting cells from a human fetus into the brain of a patient who essentially does not have a fatal condition.

CONGENITAL NERVE DISORDERS

Some children are born with nerve cells that are not coated properly by the protein called myelin. As a result, those children may have impaired function in language development and memory, and delayed motor skills seen as poor coordination and the inability to walk. The disorder has the interesting name Pelizaeus-Merzbacher disease and has no known cure. The University of San Francisco (http://neonatology.ucsf.edu/nbri/pmd-trial/) has a clinical trial open to treat these patients by direct injection of nerve stems cells into the brain. Only four patients will initially be treated. Since those nerve stem cells come from a different donor (aborted fetus), the patient has to take drugs to avoid rejection. The nerve stem cells are supplied by StemCells Inc (www.stemcellsinc.com). The same cells have already been injected into the brain of children with another congenital brain disorder called Batten disease. So far it can be concluded that the injections seem to be safe. It is too early to say whether the treatment afforded the children any benefit.

CEREBRAL PALSY

One in 100 babies suffer from this condition. Although no clinical trials are listed on the NIH trials Web site, physicians at Duke University and Northwestern University have treated children with cerebral palsy using the baby's own stored cord blood cells. Some of these kids had remarkable responses (www.msnbc.msn.com/id/23572206/), but it remains to be seen if these responses can truly be related to the infusion of cord blood cells.

To address this question, the Medical College of Georgia and Duke University are about to initiate a trial in which affected children will receive umbilical cord blood cells that were stored at birth. Half of the children will receive an infusion with saline. Since any improvements, if they happen, generally occur within three months after the infusion, patients will be assessed for any progress at that time.

MULTIPLE SCLEROSIS

This chronic disease affects the nerves and results in paralysis. Often the disease course involves phases of remission interrupted by progression. It is considered an autoimmune disease where an individual's immune system attacks his or her own cells. A clinical trial conducted at Northwestern University in Chicago recently showed that patients who were given high doses of chemotherapy and an infusion of their own bone marrow stem cells had a clear benefit. This has prompted a multicenter trial supported by the NIH conducted at different sites in the United States. The transplant team at Duke is taking a different approach: bone marrow stem cells from a tissue-matched sibling are infused after some chemotherapy is given to the patient.

MACULAR DEGENERATION

This disease of the elderly affects about fifteen million Americans. People with this disease lose central vision when delicate light-sensing cells of the macula, a region at the center of the retina, become damaged. For this trial, nerve stem cells are placed in the retina near the area of macular degeneration. These immature nerve cells produce growth factors that are believed to protect the retina cells from further damage by the disease. Although no humans have been treated as of yet, the biotech company Advanced Cell Technology has filed regulatory papers with the FDA to begin a clinical trial to treat patients with macular dystrophy in a multicenter study.

ARTHRITIS

Mesenchymal stem cells (MSC) are already approved for bone reconstruction and to support cartilage regeneration. Ongoing trials look at whether arthritis can be improved by injection of MSC into the affected join to accelerate cartilage and bone surface recovery. A ruptured ligament in the knee over time may cause arthritis in that joint as the two bones will rub against each other. Clinical trials are underway to determine if injections of MSC have any benefit.

ABOUT THE AUTHOR

Dr. Hans Klingemann is the Director of the Bone Marrow and Stem Cell Transplant Program at Tufts Medical Center in Boston and Professor of Medicine at Tufts University Medical School. He also directs the Hematological Malignancies Program at the Tufts Medical Center Cancer Center and runs a stem cell transplant research laboratory.

Dr. Klingemann has worked as a physician, scientist, educator, and administrator in leadership positions for over twenty years at various academic medical centers, has written over 150 scientific and medical papers and edited four books. He serves as editor and reviewer of several stem cell transplant journals and is a reviewer for the National Institutes of Health. He holds numerous patents and was one of the first researchers to describe the role of cord mesenchymal stem cells in transplant.